Clinical Trials Explained

A Guide to Clinical Trials
in the NHS for Healthcare
Professionals

Editors

Professor David J. Kerr
Rhodes Professor of Cancer Therapeutics and Clinical Pharmacology
Department of Clinical Pharmacology
Radcliffe Infirmary
Oxford OX2 6HE, UK

Dr Kirstine Knox
Deputy Director
National Translational Cancer Research Network
University of Oxford
Radcliffe Infirmary
Oxford OX2 6HE, UK

Diane C. Robertson
Director, Health Technology Assessment Services
ECRI Health Technology Assessment Group
5200 Butler Pike
Plymouth Meeting, PA 19462, USA

Derek Stewart
Chairman
Gedling Primary Care Trust
Byron Court
Brookfield Road
Arnold
Nottinghamshire NG5 7ER, UK

Renée Watson
Operations Manager
National Translational Cancer Research Network
University of Oxford
Radcliffe Infirmary
Oxford OX2 6HE, UK

Clinical Trials Explained

A Guide to Clinical Trials
in the NHS for Healthcare
Professionals

Produced by the British Medical Journal (BMJ),
in association with the National Translational
Cancer Research Network (NTRAC) and
ECRI (formerly the Emergency Care Research Institute)

EDITED BY

David J. Kerr

Kirstine Knox

Diane C. Robertson

Derek Stewart

Renée Watson

Blackwell
Publishing

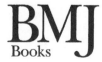

© 2006 by Blackwell Publishing Ltd
Published by Blackwell Publishing Ltd
BMJ Books is an imprint of the BMJ Publishing Group Limited, used under licence

Blackwell Publishing Inc., 350 Main Street, Malden, Massachusetts 02148-5020, USA
Blackwell Publishing Ltd, 9600 Garsington Road, Oxford OX4 2DQ, UK
Blackwell Publishing Asia Pty Ltd, 550 Swanston Street, Carlton, Victoria 3053, Australia

First published 2006

1 2006

Catalogue records for this title are available from the British Library and Library
of Congress

ISBN-13: 978-0-7279-1858-1
ISBN-10: 0-7279-1858-3

A catalogue record for this title is available from the British Library

Set in 9.5/12pt Meridien & Frutiger by TechBooks, New Delhi, India

Commissioning Editor: Mary Banks
Editorial Assistant: Mirjana Misina
Development Editor: Veronica Pock
Production Controller: Debbie Wyer

For further information on Blackwell Publishing, visit our website:
http://www.blackwellpublishing.com

The publisher's policy is to use permanent paper from mills that operate a sustainable
forestry policy, and which has been manufactured from pulp processed using acid-free
and elementary chlorine-free practices. Furthermore, the publisher ensures that the text
paper and cover board used have met acceptable environmental accreditation standards.

Clinical Trials Explained

A Guide to Clinical Trials in the NHS for Healthcare Professionals

**Produced by the British Medical Journal (BMJ),
in association with the National Translational
Cancer Research Network (NTRAC) and
ECRI (formerly the Emergency Care Research Institute)**

EDITED BY

David J. Kerr

Kirstine Knox

Diane C. Robertson

Derek Stewart

Renée Watson

Blackwell
Publishing

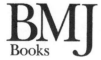

© 2006 by Blackwell Publishing Ltd
Published by Blackwell Publishing Ltd
BMJ Books is an imprint of the BMJ Publishing Group Limited, used under licence

Blackwell Publishing Inc., 350 Main Street, Malden, Massachusetts 02148-5020, USA
Blackwell Publishing Ltd, 9600 Garsington Road, Oxford OX4 2DQ, UK
Blackwell Publishing Asia Pty Ltd, 550 Swanston Street, Carlton, Victoria 3053, Australia

First published 2006

1 2006

Catalogue records for this title are available from the British Library and Library
of Congress

ISBN-13: 978-0-7279-1858-1
ISBN-10: 0-7279-1858-3

A catalogue record for this title is available from the British Library

Set in 9.5/12pt Meridien & Frutiger by TechBooks, New Delhi, India

Commissioning Editor: Mary Banks
Editorial Assistant: Mirjana Misina
Development Editor: Veronica Pock
Production Controller: Debbie Wyer

For further information on Blackwell Publishing, visit our website:
http://www.blackwellpublishing.com

The publisher's policy is to use permanent paper from mills that operate a sustainable
forestry policy, and which has been manufactured from pulp processed using acid-free
and elementary chlorine-free practices. Furthermore, the publisher ensures that the text
paper and cover board used have met acceptable environmental accreditation standards.

Contents

Preface

When the Rosetta Stone was discovered it allowed translators the first opportunity to understand Egyptian hieroglyphs, as the information carved on the stone was written in three different formats to permit as many people as possible to read and understand the text. This book provides a similar opportunity to bridge that gap between the simple patient-information-leaflet and the more complex scientific-research-orientated-text book.

First of all, I want to pay tribute to those across the research community who seek to focus their work on benefit for patients and who have taken time to write the various chapters in this book. I know, due to my own cancer experience, that it was through research that the developments in different treatments led to the improvements in my care and that of thousands of others.

As a cancer patient I found that much of the information I sought was quite simply unavailable. There were either a few introductory guides to cancer that were very basic or a large number of medical text books that were seemingly unintelligible. When I started to participate in patient involvement in cancer research I felt that, once again, there was a significant lack of relevant and substantial information about clinical trials that would strike the balance between depth and simplicity. This book provides, for the first time, to my knowledge, a collection of articles that answer the questions that many people taking part in clinical trials want to ask and receive some clarification on.

It may even encourage more people to express an interest in clinical trials, be more able to challenge and make real informed choices.

Derck C. Stewart, 2005

About ECRI

ECRI is a 40-year-old international, independent, non-profit health services research agency whose mission is to improve the quality, safety, and cost-effectiveness of healthcare through its publications, professional training and education programs, technology assessments, laboratory evaluations of medical devices, and consulting services to the healthcare community. Recognised worldwide as a trusted source of highly credible information, ECRI is designated as one of 13 Evidence-based Practice Centers in North America by the US Agency for Healthcare Research and Quality, and is a Collaborating Center of the World Health Organisation for Patient Safety, Risk Management, and Technology Assessment.

ECRI's work is distinguished by its intellectual rigor and the strict conflict-of-interest policy that governs its work. The organisation and its 300 multidisciplinary staff worldwide do not accept grants, gifts, or consulting fees from medical device or pharmaceutical companies, nor do employees or the organisation own stock in such companies. To ensure adherence to this policy, a careful auditing process examines each employee's federal income tax return after filing each year. ECRI also does not accept advertising and does not permit use of its name or its work in advertising or promotion by medical device or pharmaceutical companies.

The collective expertise at ECRI derives from its multidisciplinary staff of clinical engineers, medical technologists, doctoral level life scientists, epidemiologists, patient safety experts, occupational health safety experts, attorneys, healthcare risk managers, physicians, nurses, psychologists, medical library scientists, clinical writers and editors, and health systems consultants.

Material in this Guide is derived in large part from research ECRI performed in 2002 to produce a Guide for patients and healthcare consumers in the US considering entry into a clinical trial. That Guide, *Should I Enter A Clinical Trial?* is freely available at ECRI's US website, and is one of several patient-oriented evidence-based Guides that ECRI has developed as part of its effort to establish a National Patient Library™ of evidence-based information for patients. To develop the Guide, ECRI established a volunteer External Advisory Committee from leading US healthcare consumer and patient advocacy groups, academic institutions in the public health and health services research fields, the medical profession, industry, and government agencies. ECRI is pleased to have participated in the adaptation of this Guide for use in the UK.

Acknowledgements

The editors would like to gratefully acknowledge the contribution made by the Expert Review Committee to *Clinical Trials Explained*.

The Expert Review Committee was composed of:

- doctors, nurses and other healthcare professionals who work on clinical trials and who are known as leaders of good practice in this country and abroad;
- representatives of government and regulatory bodies concerned with ensuring clinical trials in the NHS that are conducted within the context of the international and UK ethical/legal framework; and
- patients and patient representatives with experience of participation in clinical trials.

Each member of the Expert Review Committee critically reviewed one or more drafts of *Clinical Trials Explained*. We could not have produced this guide without their thoughtful advice and unfailing support:

Professor Francine Cheater	Professor of Public Health Nursing, University of Leeds
Dr Hugh Davies	Training and Ethics Advisor, Central Office for Research Ethics Committee (COREC)
Andrea Darrington	Chair, Scarborough Patient Involvement Group
Dr Brian Dickie	Director of Research Development, Motor Neurone Disease (MND) Association
Donna Maria Fraher	Freelance consultant and patient representative for the NICE Guideline for Violent Behaviour
Elizabeth Hawkins	Radiographer and patient
U Hla Htay	Carer; Consumer Network QRD, Alzheimer's Society; consumer editor for CDCIG, Cochrane; AGPI Member, MRC; Lay Panel Member UK Human Genetic Commission
Eileen Jaffe	Chairman UK Forum, EUROPA DONNA – The European Breast Cancer Coalition
Professor Nora Kearney	Director of Cancer Care Research Centre (CCRC), Professor of Cancer Care, University of Stirling
Elizabeth Key	Patient
Jeffrey Lerner	President and Chief Executive Officer, ECRI
Dr James Mackay	Consultant Genetic Oncologist, University College London
Professor Paul Matthews	Professor of Neurology, University of Oxford

Dr Mark Middleton	Consultant Oncologist, Oxford Radcliffe NHS Trust
Richard Palmer	Carer
Ernest Parry	Chairman, Consumer Research Panel, Central South Coast Cancer Network
Cathy Ratcliffe	Senior Development and Communications Manager, National Translational Cancer Research Network (NTRAC)
Justine Smith	Deputy Director, Oncology Clinical Trials Office, University of Oxford
Dr Tony Stevens	Consumer Liaison Lead, National Cancer Research Network (NCRN)
Dr Hugh Whittall	Human Tissue Branch, Department of Health
Jenny Walton	Vulval cancer patient
Linda Ward	Clinical Study Site Manager, NTRAC
Roger Wilson	Chair, National Cancer Research Institute Consumer Liaison Group (NCRI CLG)

The editors are indebted to David Watson, Vice President of European Operations, ECRI, and Mary Banks, Publisher of BMJ Books at Blackwell Publishing without whom this guide would not have been possible.

CHAPTER 1

Overview and Purpose of this Guide to Clinical Trials in the NHS

Clinical trials are a form of medical research involving patients. They are carried out to try to find new and better ways to diagnose and treat disease. *Clinical Trials Explained* has been written as a guide for healthcare professionals seeking an introduction to clinical trials in the NHS. It aims to provide comprehensive information on why, how and what clinical trials are run in the UK. It is based on what research and discussions with patients reveal as the most critical issues that adults should understand when considering clinical trial participation. It is hoped that this guide will assist healthcare professionals when discussing care options with their patients. This chapter provides an overview of the information in this guide.

Overview and purpose of this guide

Overview

Clinical Trials Explained is a guide to clinical trials in the NHS (National Health Service). It offers carefully researched, objective information about the study of medical interventions in adult humans, and the process by which patient care is improved by comparing available and new interventions in clinical trials. Medical interventions in the context of this guide mean the:

- Diagnosis of disease, for example by using medical equipment to produce images of the diseased part of the body; and
- Treatment of disease, for example by using drugs, surgical procedures and/or medical devices such as heart pacemakers.

Please note that this guide does not address issues concerning clinical trials for preventing disease, nor does it cover clinical trials involving healthy volunteers, trials for children or trials for patients who are unconscious or not mentally able to make a decision about entering a trial.

This guide is divided into sections providing comprehensive facts about clinical trials and addressing common questions. It provides:

- An overview of clinical trials, what they are and why they are needed (Chapter 2). This chapter provides a detailed description of how clinical trials are designed and conducted, and who is involved. Chapter 2 also includes an explanation of the different trial phases, including an analysis of what each phase might mean for patients;
- A description of the process of clinical trial approval and regulation (Chapter 3). This chapter describes the organisations involved in approval and regulation, including those that pay for clinical trials and those that manage them once they are running. Chapter 3 also lists the laws and guidance used in the UK to ensure that trials are safe and of the highest quality;
- An explanation of the important concepts in clinical trials that describe design elements and research results (Chapter 4). This chapter also explains the terminology of clinical trial design and results; and
- Answers to the questions most commonly asked by patients and their carers (Chapter 5). This chapter includes information on patient rights, why patients do or do not choose to participate in clinical trials and how patients can be empowered during a clinical trial. Chapter 5 also answers important questions about the practical impact clinical trials have on their lives, e.g. costs.

This guide also provides:

- A list of additional resources providing information on how to find out about clinical trials that are available;
- A *Glossary* defining the terms used in this guide and others relating to clinical trials; and
- The ECRI Evidence Report outlining research into patients' reasons for participation in clinical trials and effect of trial participation on patient outcomes.

Purpose

The format of this guide has been developed to help the reader:

- Develop a broad understanding of clinical trials and the clinical trial process at his or her own pace;
- Find specific information of immediate importance to the reader by recognising that not all the information provided may be of interest; and
- Refer to relevant sections during discussions between patients, carers and healthcare professionals on the benefits and risks of entering a clinical trial.

Who should use this guide to clinical trials in the NHS?

This guide is for healthcare professionals, such as general practitioners and hospital doctors, research nurses and medical students, seeking an introduction to clinical trials and/or a framework for discussion with their patients about clinical trials.

Clinical Trials Explained is designed to sit alongside the patient information and decision-making tool *Clinical Trials: The Basics. Clinical Trials: The Basics* aims to provide patients with easy-to-understand information on clinical trials, as well as with simple tools to help them make a decision about whether or not to enter a clinical trial. Healthcare professionals using this guide are encouraged to make *Clinical Trials: The Basics* available to their patients to help them make informed decisions about their care. The patient guide is available via www.ecri.org.uk.

CHAPTER 2
Clinical Trials Explained

Clinical trials aim to find the best ways to diagnose and treat disease in people. Diagnostics and treatments need to be thoroughly tested in this way to ensure that the benefits to patients outweigh the risks. Thus clinical trials help to advance medical knowledge so that future patients might benefit. Clinical trials may also be of benefit to patients taking part. The team that runs a clinical trial is large, comprising:

- Scientists, doctors and other healthcare professionals;
- The organisations that pay for them;
- Those who ensure they are conducted to the highest ethical standards and abide by national and international legislation and regulatory standards; and
- Critically the patients and carers whose equal partnership is essential for success.

This chapter answers the following key questions:

- What are clinical trials?
- Why are they needed?
- Who conducts them and how are they conducted?

It also explains how clinical trials are designed, how they are conducted in phases and what the potential implications of a clinical trial are for patients.

What are clinical trials?

Scientists and doctors are continually looking to find the best ways to diagnose and treat disease. This means that they work together to:

- Develop new diagnostics and treatments and test their effects in people;
- Test a new use of an existing diagnostic or treatment in people, look at new combinations of existing treatments or change the way they are given in order to make them more effective or to reduce side effects. For example, an important radiotherapy trial showed that lung cancer patients with chest

symptoms could be treated just as effectively with two radiotherapy sessions as they could with ten sessions. This discovery has made the treatment much more convenient for patients and has reduced the potential long-term damage caused by radiotherapy;
• Compare the effectiveness of existing diagnostics and treatments in people; or
• See which diagnostics and treatments are the most cost-effective.

This form of testing is called a *clinical trial* because it scientifically tests the diagnostic or treatment in people.

Why are clinical trials needed?

Diagnostics and treatments need to be thoroughly tested in clinical trials to ensure that the benefits outweigh any risks associated with the intervention. In this context:
• *Benefit* means any positive effect on the patient's survival, quality of life and health outcomes; and
• *Risk* means fully understanding any negative impact on individuals or groups of patients.

The way benefits and risks are viewed by an individual patient is very personal. For example, a patient with Alzheimer's may consider the side effects (risk) of the best available treatment (risk) worth enduring if it means that he or she will live for as long as possible (benefit). For this patient the benefits of treatment outweigh the risks. Conversely, a cancer patient may decide that chemotherapy will reduce the quality of life significantly (risk) with only potential for small improvement in health (benefit). For this cancer patient, the risks outweigh the benefits, and hence the patient chooses not to take chemotherapy.

Clinical trials aim to understand what offers the greatest benefit to the patient with minimum risk. Both benefit and risk are carefully considered in clinical trials. Therefore clinical trials must be carried out in a controlled, methodical way so that scientists and doctors can carefully observe the effects of diagnostics and treatments being tested on patients. Thus, a clinical trial advances medical knowledge so that future patients might potentially benefit. For example, many drugs that have been tested in clinical trials are now commonly used, for example tamoxifen for breast cancer patients, and a surgical procedure called radiofrequency ablation for varicose veins. When a patient receives standard care, meaning that he or she is not involved in a clinical trial, the purpose is to benefit the individual patient only.

Clinical trial evidence is needed for interventions that are to be licensed for use in the NHS. The amount and type of evidence vary for different interventions and diseases. For example, a new cancer drug may be approved for use on the basis that it is safe. The type of cancer may not respond to currently available treatments and so the new drug may be seen as the patient's only hope. In this case a patient may decide that trying any option available outweighs the need for large amounts of clinical trial data showing how effective the drug is. This is also sometimes the case with devices like pacemakers, which are tested mainly for safety.

Who is involved in a clinical trial?

Clinical trials involve a large number of people from scientists, doctors and other front-line healthcare professionals to organisations that pay for them, organisations that ensure they are safe and conducted to the highest ethical standards and the patients without whom clinical trials would not be possible. The people involved are shown in Fig. 2.1, and are listed below:
- *the laboratory scientists* who work to understand the disease and develop new diagnostics and treatments based on this understanding;

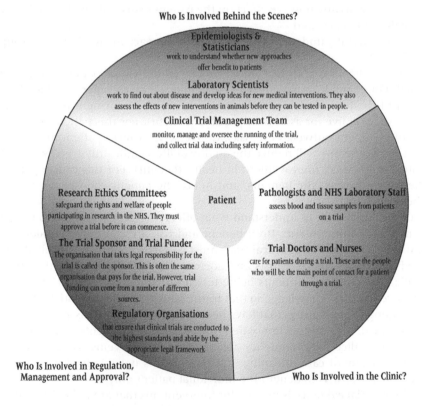

Figure 2.1 Who is involved in a clinical trial? The team that runs a clinical trial is large. It comprises: the scientists, doctors and other healthcare professionals; the organisations that pay for them; the organisations who ensure they are conducted to the highest ethical and safety standards; and critically, the patients and their carers whose equal partnership is essential for success.

- *the laboratory scientists* who work to test newly developed diagnostics and interventions in animals to assess whether they are safe and offer any potential benefit to people;
- *the front-line doctors, nurses and other healthcare professionals* who work in the NHS with patients to test diagnostics and treatments in clinical trials. These are the people who will be the main point of contact for patients in a clinical trial, and are therefore the patients' clinical trial team. The doctor, nurse and other front-line staff who work with patients participating in a clinical trial and their carers may not be the people who designed and set up the clinical trial, especially if it is a large trial with patients in many hospitals over the United Kingdom and sometimes all over the world;
- *the pathologists, medical laboratory staff and informaticians* who work to assess the effects of a medical intervention in a clinical trial by analysing, for example, patient's blood and tissue;
- *the epidemiologists, statisticians and population biologists* who work, usually in association with large clinical trials involving hundreds if not thousands of patients, to understand whether new approaches offer benefit to patients and at what risk;
- *the clinical trial management team* is made up of the management, monitoring and IT staff who coordinate and monitor hospitals and research staff, the flow of trial data, patient enrolment and safety;
- *the organisations that pay for clinical trials*, including the government, research councils, medical charities, NHS and industry that cover the costs of some £415 million estimated to take a new medical intervention from the laboratory to the clinic and the patient;
- *the trial sponsor* is the organisation that takes legal responsibility for the trial. The sponsor is often the same organisation that pays for the trial;
- *the local, national and international organisations* that ensure clinical trials are conducted to the highest ethical standards within a legal framework, and that regulate the use of new interventions in clinical trials and approve the use of new interventions in the wider population; and
- *the patients and carers*, whose equal partnership in clinical trials is essential if scientists and doctors are to make progress in the diagnosis and treatment of disease for the benefit of future generations.

In addition, a number of organisations give information about clinical trials and where they are being carried out. These are detailed under Appendix A.

How are clinical trials designed and approved?

Early laboratory work

Before a clinical trial involving patients can be planned, there must be evidence to suggest that the medical intervention shows promise. Most often this evidence is collected in the laboratory, and usually involves testing of the medical intervention in animals. The laboratory stage of development is intended to give as good an indication as possible of the potential effect of the medical intervention in people. The effect of a medical intervention in an animal is considered the best indication of what the effects are likely to be in a human. The use of animals for testing medical interventions is strictly regulated and is only allowed when strong evidence is given that no other form of testing will be adequate before proceeding to human trials.

Designing a clinical trial

Once the intervention has shown promise in the laboratory, or for a different use than it is currently being used for, the clinical trial team will agree on a key question that needs to be answered. This question is called the hypothesis. An example of a hypothesis might be:

Does heart medication significantly reduce the risk of sudden death after a heart attack?

The hypothesis and evidence already collected will determine what trial phase the intervention should be tested at. The trial phases, explained in more detail below, correspond to how much testing an intervention has already been through, with phase I as the least testing and phase IV as the most. Thus if an intervention tested in the laboratory seems it may be helpful in diagnosis or treatment, it is tested in a phase I trial. If this is successful the intervention is entered into a phase II trial and then into a phase III trial.

The team will decide what kind of patients the intervention should be tested on; this is usually based on criteria such as disease type, age, gender and how severe the disease is. These criteria are called *eligibility criteria* as they are used to determine whether or not a patient is eligible to enter a particular trial. In addition to the eligibility criteria, the team will weigh up the risks and benefits to patients to help decide which phase is the safest, and how patients will be involved. The trial team will also use statistical techniques to determine the number of patients the trial will need to recruit to maximise the certainty of the results.

In order to get clear results the trial team will set outcome measures that will be closely monitored during the trial. For example:

- Do patients on heart medication survive longer than those who do not receive the medication? The outcome measure being tested here is survival. This is a direct impact of the intervention and is called a *primary outcome measure*. At the end of the trial this will enable the trial team to say whether or not the medical intervention being tested prolongs life; and
- Do patients on heart medication feel less angina pain? The outcome measure being tested here is called a quality-of-life measure. This is an indirect impact of the intervention and is called a *secondary outcome measure*. This will enable the trial team to say whether the intervention is beneficial to patients even if it does not prolong their lives.

Seeking approval to conduct a clinical trial

Before a trial can commence, a plan, called a *clinical trial protocol* (described in Text Box 2.1), must be approved by regulatory organisations such as the

Medicines and Health Products Regulatory Agency (MHRA). These regulatory agencies use guidelines such as the International Conference on Harmonisation guidance on Good Clinical Practice (ICH-GCP) to decide whether a trial is of high enough quality and safety to go ahead. The clinical trial protocol together with the *patient information sheet* and the *patient consent form* must be approved by national and local research ethics committees (RECs) to ensure that the trial is conducted to the highest ethical standards. Further information on clinical trial regulation and ethical approval can be found in Chapter 3.

Text Box 2.1: What is a clinical trial protocol?

Every clinical trial is based on a detailed plan. The plan includes a variety of information on:
- How the trial will be run;
- The scientific evidence to support the trial;
- Eligibility criteria; and
- Which outcomes will be measured.

The plan is referred to as the trial protocol. The protocol contains all the information needed to prepare, conduct and conclude the trial. The protocol is one of the documents that will go to the ethics committee and regulatory authorities for approval.

Progression of a medical intervention through the clinical trial phases

Generally, clinical trials are divided into four phases. Each phase acts as a checkpoint, where testing is not allowed to progress to the next phase unless sufficient evidence is collected to support further testing. Regulatory and ethical approval must also be gained before a medical intervention can progress to the next phase. Figure 2.2 and the information below outline the four clinical trial phases.

Phase I is the earliest stage of testing when a medical intervention is either:
- Being tested in people for the first time. The primary aim of this type of phase I trial is to test safety; or
- Already being used in the NHS in a specific way but is being considered for a new use. This type of trial aims to find out if the intervention is effective for a different disease, at a different dose or administration method.

A medical intervention approved for testing in a phase I trial must have very good laboratory evidence to show that toxicity is understood.

Phase II trials proceed after a medical intervention is shown to be acceptably safe in a phase I trial. Phase II trials involve more participants, so a better understanding of the safety can be gained and the team can begin to assess how effective the intervention may be.

early stage of development, no evidence has accumulated in humans indicating that the treatment will be effective. Several published articles that have reviewed the therapeutic outcomes of patients in phase I cancer trials have found that the actual therapeutic benefit in these trials ranges from 3–5% of patients.

Sometimes a phase I trial is offered to a patient as a 'last hope' because no other treatment has worked and a doctor has no other standard treatment to offer. Hope is very important. It is also natural for patients to want to try anything available and for their doctors to want to offer something else, especially if the patient wants to undergo more treatment. As the husband of a cancer patient said,

> *Even if the doctors had told us she had only a 1% chance of benefit, we would have done the trial. She was young, we had children, and she wanted to take any chance at all.*

Phase I trials are extremely important in these situations – and the patients who enter them are benefiting future patients by helping to advance medical knowledge. In most cases these trials are the only way that new medical interventions can be developed. If patient expectations are high for health improvement in a phase I trial, patients and their carers may feel very disappointed when it does not happen. The risks are generally greater in early-phase trials and so patients may want to consider the potential impact of a phase I trial on their quality of life (such as treatment side effects, time commitment and travel requirements) and how they want to spend their remaining time.

So before a patient agrees to enter a phase I study, he or she should understand that these trials carry the least potential for benefit and the greatest potential for risk of side effects because the only evidence at this point is from animal or laboratory studies or from results of the treatment for some other disease. A patient's experience of an early-phase clinical trial is given in Text Box 2.2.

Text Box 2.2: An American patient's experience of an early-phase trial

My wife, Maria was 40 years old, athletic, and very fit, but a heavy smoker. One cold January day she started to feel a 'wheeze' in her chest, which increasingly became stronger, and went to see our family doctor. Chest x-rays showed a shadow that made him believe that she had an infection. He prescribed antibiotics, but she didn't feel any better. A few weeks later, the doctor ordered a computed tomography (CT) scan of her chest. It detected a 'mass'. A biopsy revealed that she had advanced non-small-cell lung cancer. We went to doctors at a renowned cancer centre. They told us the tumour's location made it impossible to remove by surgery. The only option was a very aggressive series of radiation treatments. Because of her relative youth and otherwise good health, the doctors went 'for the cure'. She underwent 30 radiation sessions. Very shortly after some initial relief, her condition deteriorated from all the undesirable side effects of treatment.

Maria carried an oxygen tank for more than three months to help her breathe. She never showed desperation, never complained. Not even during those long nights when she was coughing without relief. One Monday, after a terrible night and against her will, I called her doctor. He asked me to take her and meet him at Accident and Emergency. Once there, he said, 'Maria, I have to treat you, and the only chance that you may have is Taxol, an experimental drug that has been successfully used for other types of cancer. It is now being tried for non-small-cell tumours like yours. There is still not much data about it'.

It was an early-phase trial. The doctor explained to us that the patients would be randomly assigned to different types of drugs. We didn't ask too many questions. We were afraid, but we explained the situation to our two daughters (then 9 and 14 years old). I told my wife that the decision had to be hers, but I would give my opinion if she wanted it. I told her that most of all I was going to support her, whatever her decision. She decided to enrol in the trial. She wanted any chance at survival. We were happy to learn that she had been assigned to the group to be treated with the maximum doses of Taxol. Although we knew there was almost no chance, my wife, our girls, and I never lost hope. She recovered slightly after her first treatment, but two days before the second session she started to cough heavily. I took her to accident and emergency again.

Soon after, they began her second round of Taxol, but it had to be interrupted. She was put on a respirator. The heavy cough seemed to come from her 'good' lung. An emergency biopsy revealed that her other lung was compromised too.

As I write these words on the eighth anniversary of my wife's death, I ask myself if we did the 'right' thing. The answer is absolutely yes. On the other hand, I ask myself if I would make the same decision if I had to go through that one more time? I don't know. We did what we felt was right at the time.

Taxol is now used in combination with other drugs as standard treatment for a number of cancers.

Phase II clinical trials

By the time a medical intervention reaches phase II, the clinical trial team will know quite a lot about it. The phase I trial must show what the risks are likely to be for patients and whether there are any signs that the intervention has any positive effect or benefit. The main purpose of a phase II trial is to study efficacy and further refine the optimal drug dose, device use or procedure technique. The likelihood of individual health improvement is still limited in a phase II trial and the effects of the intervention are closely measured to see if the patient's health improves.

A phase II trial may be the first time a patient will come across the concept of a *controlled trial* and random assignment to a group. Most often, a patient will be assigned to one of two different groups: the trial group and the control group. The trial group receives the intervention being tested. The control group receives a comparable standard intervention or an inactive form of the intervention. The allocation of patients to groups is done by random assignment, called *randomisation*. Randomisation is a scientific method of assigning patients to different groups in a trial so that valid results can be obtained. Randomisation and controlled trials are explained in more detail in Chapter 4.

In a phase II trial, the criteria used to determine patient eligibility (inclusion and exclusion criteria) are usually more specific than those in phase I. In phase II, the patients usually have similar medical characteristics and the same medical condition. As with any phase of trial, the trial protocol should help clarify any questions that arise. Phase II trials typically take several months to several years to complete (depending on what is being studied). Phase II trials include more patients than phase I trials – usually from 50 to a few hundred patients.

Phase III clinical trials

On the basis of positive results from earlier phase trials, the researchers will design a protocol for a phase III trial. Again, regulatory organisations will assess the trial protocol. The REC for the NHS Trust conducting the trial must approve the protocol before the trial can proceed. The possible benefits and risks of the treatment are better defined by phase III – but are still not entirely known.

The main purpose of a phase III trial is usually to compare the effectiveness and safety of the trial intervention with an intervention currently being used for the disease. It is hoped that one of the interventions will be found to be more effective, or equally as effective but with fewer side effects. Phase III trials clarify the efficacy, best doses and routes of administration of a drug and optimal settings and performance characteristics of a device. These trials also provide the opportunity to identify less common side effects because they typically enrol hundreds to thousands of patients and may last several months to several years. Phase III trials usually include control groups and use of randomisation procedures for assigning patients to groups. Phase III may also include *blinding*, which means not revealing to patients and/or researchers which treatment group a patient is in. These terms are explained in detail in Chapter 4.

On completion of a phase III trial of a new medical intervention, the clinical trial team will aim to have gathered enough information for the medical intervention to be considered for standard use in the NHS. All the information gathered will be sent to the MHRA that will consider whether a license should be issued for use in the NHS.

A patient can enter a phase III trial with more expectation than in earlier phase trials of a possible therapeutic benefit; however, efficacy is still not well established and not all risks have been identified. For example, if a drug is going to cause a rare adverse event – meaning that the event may happen only once in every 1000 patients who get the drug – it may only be seen after a large number of people have received the drug. Also, even if the intervention has some efficacy, not all patients may respond. So, there is a chance of receiving little or no therapeutic benefit in a phase III trial, even if the intervention has been shown to work in other patients. A patient's experience of a phase III trial can be found in Text Box 2.3.

Text Box 2.3: A patient's experience of a phase III trial

I was on a phase III trial. It was offered to me because I had an inoperable tumour and chemotherapy was the only treatment option available. The options were to enter the trial, or to have chemotherapy outside the trial. As a result I did not feel like a guinea pig. I felt a bit special in fact – as I was randomised onto the only arm of the trial which called for in-patient treatment. I was glad about that. From the patient information sheet, I automatically did what I expect everyone does, decided which of the trial arms I would like to be treated on, even though I realised there was only a 1 in 3 chance of getting it. I got it, I was glad to get it and felt a greater degree of commitment to the trial as a result.

The protocol called for 72-hour continuous infusion of the experimental drug. During the seemingly endless days in hospital, twice my night-time change of drug (3 changes a day for three days) got lost. I was worried that would distort trial data, and had to be reassured it wouldn't. The extra visits for blood tests (done by my GP) were not to be missed – I was disciplined about ensuring that the protocol (of which I had a copy) was followed.

The treatment was thrice-weekly doses for six cycles – almost four months with periods of nausea, tiredness and generally feeling fragile. I was fortunate not to have too many side-effects – a result of being quite fit and active to within a few weeks of starting the trial. Possibly the worst part of the experience was the sense of isolation when I was in hospital. The nursing staff were always busy, I had occasional visits from the research sister, a daily visit from the SHO, and my oncologist came round once during each stay. The other memorable part of the treatment was that England beat West Indies in a test series that summer, and I was able to listen, largely undisturbed, to great swathes of Test Match Special.

I am fortunate to have been in a poor prognosis group and to be in remission. The trial gave me access to a drug I would not have had as standard first-line treatment, although it is the second-line treatment. I continue to have a sense of ownership of the trial, even after more than four years, and am looking forward, with some trepidation to the eventual publication of the final trial results.

Phase IV clinical trials

A phase IV study may be conducted after a medical intervention has been licensed for use in the NHS by the MHRA. These are usually large studies and are sometimes required as a condition of licensing a new treatment. Phase IV trials may aim to:

- See how well the treatment works in a broader mix of patients and to assess the effect on factors such as quality of life;
- Gain more information about side effects and their frequency – especially ones that were serious but not seen too often in smaller, earlier phase trials;
- Develop new uses for the intervention;
- Assess the cost effectiveness and implications of the intervention; and
- Compare one intervention with a competitor's to see if it has any clinical advantages.

By phase IV, risks are much better defined and a body of evidence on efficacy has accumulated. An example of a phase IV study can be found in Text Box 2.4.

Text Box 2.4: Example of a phase IV clinical trial

GlaxoSmithKline conducted a phase IV trial of commonly used asthma medications. Currently people with severe long-term asthma may take high doses of steroid asthma inhalers every day. The trial aimed to compare two different inhalers. One inhaler contained a combination of two medicines and the other only one medicine. The plan was to see if one inhaler allowed patients to reduce the use of inhaled steroid without losing control of their asthma. In this trial the patients were too severely asthmatic to achieve sufficient control to see a difference between the two inhalers. However it helped provide information about how other trials could be designed to examine possible ways of reducing the long-term side effects of treatment and possibly improve the patients' quality of life.

This trial was conducted in 34 medical centres across 10 countries.

Overviews and meta-analyses

Clinical trials contribute to medical knowledge, and like a jigsaw puzzle each trial represents a piece of the big picture. In order to fully understand what the big picture looks like, the data from all trials on a particular disease or intervention are compiled and analysed. This type of analysis can be achieved by conducting an overview study or meta-analysis. Overviews and meta-analyses use complex statistics and analytical methods to pool data from patients across multiple clinical trials. The results of an overview or meta-analysis help clarify what works and in whom it works best because an entire body of data from many trials is analysed. Overviews and meta-analyses do not involve patients directly, but because they assess multiple trials, the data comes from the hundreds of thousands of patients who have participated in trials, usually involving many countries.

Summary

This chapter of the guide sets out to answer the following questions:
- *What are clinical trials?* Clinical trials involve the testing of medical interventions in people. Clinical trials are carried out in a controlled, methodical way so that scientists and doctors can carefully observe the effects of diagnostics and treatments on patients. The main aim of a clinical trial is to advance medical knowledge for the benefit of future patients.
- *Why are they needed?* Clinical trials are needed to provide an environment where the benefits and risk of a medical intervention can be measured objectively. Clinical trials are the best known way to carefully measure and compare the safety and efficacy of medical interventions.
- *Who is involved in clinical trials?* There are many individuals and organisations involved in clinical trials, including those who design and conduct them, e.g. laboratory scientists and the clinical trial team including front-line doctors, nurses and other healthcare professionals; those who monitor and manage the trial (scientists involved in assessing information from clinical trials such as blood and clinical data, and clinical trial management teams); organisations that pay for clinical trials; organisations involved in regulation and approval of trials; and critical patients and their carers.
- *How are clinical trials designed and approved?* Clinical trials are designed based on results from the laboratory and previous clinical research. Each clinical trial is developed into two important documents that are needed to decide whether or not a trial should be approved; they are:
  - The clinical trial protocol, which is a detailed plan of the trial. The clinical trial protocol outlines, for example, details of the medical intervention that will be tested, the evidence to support the trial, the questions that the trial aims to answer and the outcomes that will be measured; and
  - The patient information sheet, which is a summary of the trial protocol. The patient information sheet is intended to give patients information that will help them decide whether they want to, or are eligible to, participate in the trial.
- *How are clinical trials conducted?* Clinical trials are divided into four phases. The phases correspond to how much is already known about the medical intervention:
  - Phase I trial: the earliest stage of testing. Most phase I trials involve the testing of new medical interventions that have never been tested in people before, so the risks are highest and chance of benefit is only 3–5%. These trials test the safety and dose of the intervention in small numbers of people (10–20);
  - Phase II trial: the next stage of testing. The effects of the medical intervention on the disease can begin to be tested. Phase II trials involve

testing of interventions for safety and efficacy in larger numbers of people (50–200);

– Phase III trial: phase III trials usually test whether the trial intervention is any better than an intervention currently used in the NHS. The main risks are well understood by this stage and there is a greater potential for benefit. By including hundreds, if not thousands of patients, these trials find out about less common side effects; data from phase III trials are submitted to obtain licensing for a drug or device;

– Phase IV trial: this is the final stage of testing and may be required as a condition of licensing approval. The trial involves hundreds to thousands of patients. Phase IV trials aim to get a better understanding of a medical intervention after it has been licensed. Information may be gathered on rarer side effects, better dosage and cost effectiveness.

CHAPTER 3
Clinical Trial Approval, Regulation and Funding

Clinical trials are strictly regulated at all stages. This Chapter considers the steps that need to be taken and the organisations involved in getting the go ahead to run a clinical trial. The regulation of clinical trials is important to ensure that the trials that are run are scientifically valuable, are as safe as possible and have the greatest chance of improving patient care.

Clinical trials are extremely expensive to run, and there are strict legal obligations for the organisation that takes responsibility for the trial. Therefore funding organisations and organisations taking legal responsibilities are critical to the smooth running and success of a trial. This Chapter aims to explain all the organisations involved in approving, regulating and funding a clinical trial run in the NHS in the UK.

How are clinical trials approved and regulated?

Clinical trials run in the NHS are conducted according to European Law and Guidance, which has been tailored for the UK. These regulatory requirements make up the UK Research Governance Framework. A number of organisations take part in the approval and regulatory processes required under the Research Governance Framework. Text Box 3.1 describes the organisations involved, and Figure 3.1 sets out the recommended process by which clinical trials and developed and approved.

Ethical approval

The approval and regulatory organisations, as well as the clinical trial team, work to a set of guidance and laws set out in a number of important documents. Text Box 3.2 lists the main documents that are used to regulate UK clinical trials and how to find out more about them.

Text Box 3.1: Organisations and processes involved in the trial approval process

Medicines and Healthcare Products Regulatory Agency (MHRA): The MHRA protects and promotes public health and patient safety by ensuring that medicines, healthcare products and medical equipment meet appropriate standards of safety, quality, performance and effectiveness.

Local NHS Research and Development Committees: Each NHS Trust has a Research and Development Committee (R&D Committee). The R&D Committee is responsible for assessing and approving clinical trials that will run in their NHS Trust. The R&D Committee are part of the Department of Health.

The Trial Sponsor: Every trial must have an individual, company, institution or organisation that takes legal responsibility for the trial. Often the Sponsor is the same as the funding body, but not always.

The Trial Funding Body: Funding for trials normally comes from industry, a charity or a Research Council. Because of the high cost of trials, it is becoming more common for funding to be obtained from a number of organisations.

Peer Review: This is a process where a panel of scientists and healthcare professionals who are not involved with the trial assess the trial protocol for scientific and medical quality. Usually the organisation that is funding or sponsoring the trial will have an independent system for peer review.

Central Office of Research Ethics Committees (COREC): COREC safeguards the rights, dignity and welfare of people participating in research in the NHS. COREC coordinates all the Research Ethics Committees (REC) around the UK. The REC must review and give approval before any clinical trial can proceed. REC members must have no personal connection with the trial. They can be patients, members of the public, nurses, doctors, statisticians, pharmacists and academics, as well as people with specific ethical expertise gained through a legal, philosophical or theological background.

European Medicines Agency (EMEA): This is a body of the European Union with headquarters in London. Its main responsibility is the protection and promotion of public and animal health. The EMEA coordinates the evaluation and supervision of human and veterinary medicinal products throughout the European Union.

What is the role of an ethics committee in regulation?

In addition to their main role in approving clinical trials, research ethics committees (RECs) automatically receive a quarterly and annual report on each clinical trial they have approved. These reports provide an update on the progress of the trial, particularly the safety information that has been gathered, and a report from the trial data monitoring committee. The final report

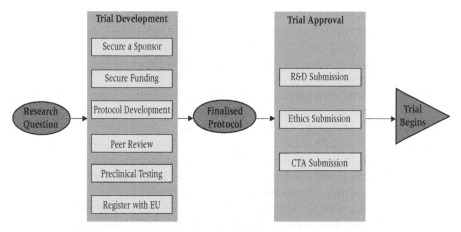

Figure 3.1 How are clinical trials developed and approved? This figure sets out the recommended process, in line with the requirements of the UK Research Governance Framework, by which clinical trials are developed and approved.

a REC will receive is called an 'end of trial' report. The end of trial report includes the results of the trial and a summary of what has been learned.

Text Box 3.2: Guidance and laws used to regulate clinical trials

EU Clinical Trials Directives (2001/20/EC) is the latest European regulations on clinical trials. This aims to harmonise the clinical trial standards used across Europe (http://www.wcth.org.uk/downloads/EU Directive/Directive.pdf)

Medicines for Human Use (Clinical Trials) Regulations (S12004/1031) is the UK law on regulation of clinical trials, which is being used to implement the EU Directive on Clinical Trials, (http://www.legislation. hmso.gov.uk/si/si2004/20041031.htm)

Research Governance Framework reflects a wide range of discussions with the NHS and all the Department of Health's partners in health and social care research. (http://www.dh.gov.uk/assetRoot/04/01/47/57/ 04014757.pdf)

Central Office for Research Ethics Committee (COREC) provides guidance on how to apply for ethical review for any trial in the United Kingdom other then gene therapy trials.COREC guidance sets out what a clinical trial should provide for patients. (http://www.corec.org.uk/)

Gene Therapy Advisory Committee is the national research ethics committee for all clinical trials involving genr therapy. (www.advisorybodies.doh.gov.uk/genetics/gtac/)

Continued

European Clinical Trials Database is a database where every trial in Europe must be listed (https://eudract.emea.eu.int/eudract/index/.do).
Registration with EUDRACT will result in :
– A EUDRACT number being allocated; this is required for clinical trial approval; and
– A clinical trial application being prepared; this will be submitted to the regulatory organisations.
Declaration of Helsinki is a statement of ethical principles developed in 1964 by the world Medical Association, and updated most recently in 2004. The Declaration of Helsinki provides guidance on ethical issues for people designing and conducting clinical trials, and people involved in clinical trials. (http:// www.wma.net/e/policy/b3.htm)
Nuremberg Code was devloped after the second world war to ensure that people were not forced to participate in research. The Nuremberg code states that voluntary consent is absolutely essential in order for a research project to be conducted.
International Conference on Harmonisation guidance on Good Clinical Practice (ICH-GCP) is a set of guidelines recognised across the world for running clinical trials. The ICH-GCP guidelines ensure patient safety, data quality and that trials are conducted to the highest standards. (http://www.ich.org)

How do we ensure that ethics committees are doing a good job?

COREC is introducing a system of assessing the quality of RECs. This will involve introducing 'ghost applications' to the system and monitoring of progress and outcome of ethical review.

Informed consent

A patient must give his or her written permission, or consent, to be entered into a clinical trial. Participation is entirely voluntary. Consent must be given without any direct or indirect coercion or inducement. Therefore, patients must be given sufficient information orally and in writing about the clinical trial, in the language and a format they understand, to enable them to exercise their right to make an informed decision about whether or not to participate.

This process is based on the principle that people have the right to be informed of all the possible known benefits and risks of taking part in the trial, because they are considering volunteering for an experiment. This right is enshrined in UK law in line with international guidelines; further details on the legal framework within which clinical trials are conducted are given in Chapter 5.

If a patient decides to take part in a clinical trial, he or she will be asked to sign a *consent form* and retain a copy. The patient receives a copy of the consent form because it contains important information that he or she may want or need to refer to during the trial. This process of discussion and giving permission in writing is known as *informed consent*.

Various guidelines have been drawn up on what information people need in order to consent to or to decline taking part in a clinical trial. But there is a lot of discussion about what people really want to know and, of course, this varies from person to person. Research into this issue is considered in greater detail in Text Box 3.3.

Text Box 3.3: An example of research into factors contributing to patient understanding

A published study of 207 cancer patients who enroled in phase I or phase II clinical trials in three medical centres in the United States looked at patient understanding of the trials after completing the consent process. It was found that less than 40% of the patients who enrolled realised that receiving an experimental treatment might increase their risk or discomfort compared to standard treatments. However, virtually all patients were highly satisfied with the consent process. This study noted several things that contributed to greater patient understanding:

• Reading consent forms and patient information sheets carefully;
• Having a nurse present during discussions about the clinical trial;
• Taking the time to consider the participation decision carefully by taking the consent form and patient information sheet home overnight; and
• Receiving a simplified consent form.

Joffe S, Cook EF, Cleary PD, Clark JW, Weeks JC. Quality of informed consent in cancer clinical trials: a cross-sectional survey. Lancet 24 Nov 2001.

What really matters is that the patients are satisfied and have enough information and time to make an informed decision about what is right for them as an individual. Patients should not sign a consent form if they do not feel comfortable with the information given or if they do not feel they fully understand the benefits and risks. To help a patient decide whether he or she wants to take part or not, the trial doctor or nurse should:

• Discuss the trial and any alternatives to entering the trial with the patient. Patients should feel free to ask any questions they believe are important in helping them reach a decision. The clinical trial doctor or nurse who participates in this discussion should be knowledgeable about the study and be able to answer all the patient's questions;
• Encourage the patients to explain in their own words what they think the trial is about to them, how long they will be in the trial, what the risks and benefits are, what is not known and how trial-related complications might

be dealt with should they arise. This will help the patient and clinical trial doctor or nurse appreciate how well the information is understood. It also helps to empower the patient by taking responsibility and control of his or her involvement in the trial. In addition, if they wish, patients should be able to bring a family member or friend with whom they can discuss options with afterwards. The trial doctor or nurse should feel confident that the patient understands the information and his or her options;

- Give the patient a copy of the *consent form* together with written information about the trial – called a *patient information sheet* – to be read at leisure. Text Box 3.4 shows what should be included in a patient information sheet, and Text Box 3.5 provides a checklist of what should be covered by the consent form. This allows the patient the opportunity to discuss trial participation with family or friends. It also helps the people who will be supporting the patient through the trial to understand more about what is required;
- Allow the patient as much time as he or she needs to make a decision on participating. However, for some trial the patient eligibility criteria stipulate that a patient must enter a clinical trial within a certain time frame. The clinical trial doctor or nurse should make this time frame clear without pressuring an uncertain patient.

The trial doctor and nurse should continue to provide information to the patient as the patient or the situation requires during the trial. Consent forms and patient information sheets should be updated with new information, when appropriate.

Text Box 3.4: Patient information sheet

Every trial must provide an information sheet designed primarily for patients and their carers. The patient information sheet outlines all the information that a patient should need to be able to make an informed decision about whether they want to participate in a trial. The main features of a patient information sheet include:

- A summary of the clinical trial protocol in language that is clear and concise and easy to understand (provided in a language other than English if needed);
- A list of the characteristics that the clinical trial team need patients to meet in order to participate;
- A statement of the known and potential benefits and risks to patients; and
- An outline of what will be expected of a participant. For example what medical tests will be required and how much time the patient will need to spend receiving the trial intervention.

The patient information sheet will be carefully examined by the ethics committee and is an essential part of the approval process.

Text Box 3.5: Checklist: What should a consent form and patient information sheet include?

This checklist can help assess whether a consent form and patient information sheet contains all the kinds of information they should. This is based on guidance provided by COREC to researchers planning to conduct a clinical trial. It includes the principles of the International Conference on Harmonisation guidance on Good Clinical Practice (ICH-GCP) guidelines. The patient information sheet and consent form should include:

- The trial title – this should be understandable;
- An invitation to participate in the trial – a statement that the trial involves research;
- The purpose of the trial – the background and aim of the trial together with the duration of the trial;
- Who is funding and organising the clinical trial;
- A description of how the trial was approved and which organisations have been involved;
- An outline of the role and rights of the patient;
- An explanation of how the participants are chosen and how many participants will be studied;
- A statement confirming that taking part in the research is entirely voluntary;
- An explanation of what is expected of patients and what will happen to them, e.g. time needed for treatment;
- Information about potential expense reimbursement if more frequent visits are required to clinic;
- A basic description of the drug or device including the stage of development, dose and administration;
- An explanation of possible side effects, including for trials involving new drugs, a statement explaining that there may be unknown side effects;
- A description of foreseeable benefits and risks or discomfort to participants, e.g. in the case of pregnancy;
- Information about what will happen if a previously unknown condition is discovered during the trial;
- A statement regarding private health insurance, e.g. if a patient discovers that he or she has high blood pressure;
- Disclosure of appropriate alternative procedures or sources of treatment that might be available;
- A statement about how information that may become available during the trial will be communicated;
- A statement about what will happen at the end of the study;

Continued

- The policy for dealing with complaints and details about what redress may be available;
- Assurances of confidentiality should medical records need to be accessed;
- A statement that the participant's general practitioner will be notified of his or her participation in the trial.

How are trials managed?

Once a clinical trial has been approved, the same organisations set out in Text Box 3.1 will work with the clinical trial management team to regulate the trial. Regulation involves the following:

- *Safety reporting:* This requires the clinical trial management team to record, notify, assess, report, analyse and manage adverse events in the trials they are managing. Adverse events are occasions when a patient has a negative experience related to the trial. The degree of severity of the side effect is measured as:
  - an adverse event (AE);
  - a serious adverse event (SAE);
  - serious adverse reaction (SAR); and
  - suspected unexpected serious adverse reaction (SUSAR).
- *Progress reporting:* The trial management team is required to provide regular updates on how the trial is progressing. This includes whether there have been any adverse events. The progress report will be sent to the regulatory organisations, REC, funding body or bodies and sponsor, and the clinical trial doctors.
- *Management and monitoring:* Ongoing management and monitoring of the trial is needed to ensure that standards are met and patients are safe. This involves the review of safety data as they are reported and regular review of the overall trial data. Monitoring of data can also be done by trial staff visiting hospitals to check data forms against patient notes. This ensures that data have been reported correctly and that patients are on the correct treatment.
- *MHRA inspection:* The MHRA is responsible for ensuring that the trial sponsor is working to the correct standards. This is a legal requirement, so all trial management offices must be inspected by the MHRA to be able to manage trials. Other regulatory organisations may also conduct inspections.
- *Audit:* Regulatory organisations, funding bodies and sponsors may want to conduct an audit of the place where the clinical trial will take place. R&D offices will be auditing research in their organisation as part of their responsibilities under Research Governance Framework.
- *Urgent safety measures:* If an adverse event occurs or in any other emergency situation, the trial management team must contact the MHRA and REC, who will decide whether or not the trial is safe to proceed. The trial doctor

can change trial procedures if a patient is in immediate danger. Any such changes must be reported to the MHRA and REC as soon as possible.

Who pays for a clinical trial?

Funding for clinical trials will most often come from one or more of the following sources:

- *Industry*: The pharmaceutical and biotechnology industries allocate significant funding for clinical trials;
- *Research councils:* Research councils such as the Medical Research Council allocate government funds for the conduct of a variety of research including clinical trials; and
- *Charities*: The UK is very fortunate to have a strong charitable sector that actively funds a large number of clinical trials.

Increasingly multiple funding bodies are working together to cover the costs of trials. For example a charity and a pharmaceutical company will often form partnerships to make sure that trials are properly funded and run as well as possible. Trials are normally either:

- *Academic-led*, where the Chief Investigator (CI) is a health professional working for the NHS. The CI will submit the proposal to a funding body for scientific review and overall assessment; or
- *Industry-led*, where a company will approach a well-established academic investigator to conduct the research on its behalf, whilst taking overall responsibility for the trial.

Both academic- and industry-led research undergo very rigorous assessment on scientific, clinical and ethical quality. The role of investigators and their relationships with funding bodies should be clearly stated during the trial approval process. It is increasingly common for academics to work closely and have good working relationships with companies; this helps the field of research enormously. However, in order to ensure that the research is conducted without bias, conflicts of interest must be declared.

Summary

This chapter looks in more detail at the approval and regulatory processes involved in getting a clinical trial started and running including:

How clinical trials are approved and regulated including ethical requirements – Clinical trials in the UK must run according to the legal and ethical standards set out in the Research Governance Framework. This involves:

- Multiple regulatory organisations including:
  - Medicines and Health Products Regulatory Agency (MHRA)
  - Local NHS Research and Development committees
  - The trial sponsor
  - The trial funding body

- Research Ethics Committees (RECs)
- European Medicines Agency (EMEA)
- Multiple regulatory and legal documents including:
  - EU Clinical Trials Directive
  - Medicines for Human Use (Clinical Trials) Regulations (S12004/1031)
  - Research Governance Framework
  - Central Office for Research Ethics Committee (COREC)
  - Gene Therapy Advisory Committee (GTAC)
  - European Clinical Trials database that issue a EUDRACT number and a clinical trial application;
  - Declaration of Helsinki – a statement of ethical principals to provide guidance to people designing and conducting clinical trials, and people involved in clinical trials;
  - Nuremberg Code – outlines the requirement for all research participants to give voluntary consent; and
  - International Conference on Harmonisation guidance on Good Clinical Practice (ICH-GCP)

The process of ensuring that patients have a good understanding of what a trial might mean for them before giving consent– Every clinical trial requires two important, ethically regulated documents for patients: The patient information sheet that provides a clear outline of what the trial involves; and the consent form which a patient must sign before he or she enters a clinical trial and only after being sure he or she understands the information received.

How trials are managed – The clinical trial management team works with the MHRA, Research Ethics Committees and local R&D committees to manage the running of the trial and to monitor safety. Regular updates are also required from the funding bodies and sponsor.

Who pays for clinical trials – Clinical trials are usually funded by a company, a charity of medical research council. The high cost of trials means that trials are increasingly being paid for through a collaboration of fuding bodies.

CHAPTER 4
Understanding Clinical Trial Design and Results

This chapter of the guide looks at concepts primarily associated with phase II and phase III trials including randomisation, blinding, controlled trials and placebo.

These concepts describe the way a clinical trial is designed and run. They have significant implications on what a patient can expect during a clinical trial. For example, randomisation is the process by which patients are assigned to a group in a trial where they receive either standard treatment (control), an inactive form of the treatment (placebo) or an active test intervention. Before patients can decide whether they want to enter a trial that uses randomisation, it will be important for them to understand that they may not receive the test intervention. This may effect their decision to enter.

This chapter also explains the language used to describe the results of a clinical trial. For a patient participating in a clinical trial, words such as partial response (the disease is improving) or stable (there is no change in disease), may be some of the most important words he or she hears. These words describe whether their disease is being affected by the test intervention.

Understanding randomisation and blinding in clinical trials

In most phase III and some phase II trials, a computer is used to assign a patient to the arm of a trial where he or she receives standard treatment (control), an inactive form of the treatment (placebo) or the test intervention. This scientific process is called *randomisation*. For an individual patient, randomisation determines which group of the trial he or she is in:

- *The test group:* Patients randomised to the test treatment group receive the trial diagnostic or treatment that is being tested alone or in combination with other interventions in the clinical trial; or

- *The control group:* Patients randomised to the control group receive an intervention against which the clinical trial team can measure the effects of the test intervention. A patient assigned to the control group will receive:
- The current standard diagnostic or treatment used in the NHS at the time – this may be to 'watch and wait,' for example in some trials for prostate cancer patients; or
- An 'inactive' form of the treatment; this is called a *placebo*.

Without a control group it is impossible to measure whether any benefit seen in the trial is due to the test intervention or other factors not related to the test treatment. Controls and placebos are discussed in detail in the following section of this chapter.

The process of randomisation was developed as early as the 1940s (see Text Box 4.1) to overcome issues affecting the validity of the clinical trial results. Randomisation aims to help ensure that the results seen are due to the treatment given. Patients entering a trial are allocated to a trial group by a computer that makes sure that different patient characteristics are evenly

---

Text Box 4.1: The first reported randomised clinical trial: effective treatment for TB

In the early 1940s encouraging results from trials on a small number of patients suggested that the new antibiotic streptomycin might be effective for treating an often-fatal condition, pulmonary tuberculosis (TB). The drug, made by a US manufacturer, was not readily available in the UK, and doctors did not welcome the responsibility of deciding which TB patients should and should not get a *promising but not yet proven* new drug.

To try to find out how well the new drug really worked and on whom, two British doctors designed what is thought to be one of the first truly randomised controlled trials. Randomisation, a new concept, determined who would get the experimental drug. The trial tested the new antibiotic against the standard care of the day in the UK – bed rest. No placebo was given because doctors felt it would be too painful (several injections daily) for patients not actually receiving the experimental drug.

Ninety-seven patients with severe TB were randomly assigned to receive either the drug injections or hospital bed rest. Neither doctors nor patients knew beforehand which treatment a particular patient was going to receive. The results published in 1948 in the *British Medical Journal* showed that 51% of the 55 patients in the treatment group had significant improvement after six months compared to only 8% of 52 patients in the bed rest group.

Streptomycin went on to become a proven standard of care in the UK, US, and elsewhere.

and randomly distributed among the control and test treatment groups. This process ensures that each group contains similar numbers of patients with similar characteristics. At its simplest, this means that the gender or ages of patients will be the same in each group of the trial. However, it is more likely that the patient's medical history, previous treatments and current state of health are also taken into consideration when ensuring patients are enroled evenly into the different trial groups.

Typically, a letter or number is used to designate each test group, and patients are identified by a code of some sort – often a number. In the case of clinical trials of new treatments, the treatment given to patients in each group appears identical so that no one – usually neither the doctor nor the patient – can tell whether a patient is receiving the active test intervention or a control intervention or placebo. This is called *blinding* or *masking*. There are two types of blinding:

- A *single-blind trial* is where the patient does not know which test group he or she has been assigned to. The front-line healthcare professionals on the clinical trial team will know which group the patient has been assigned to; and
- A *double-blind trial* is where neither the patient nor the trial doctor knows which group the patient has been assigned to. In the case of a drug treatment trial, the patient's doctor will be issued with a computer-coded treatment pack, and only by breaking the computer code can the identity of the drug or placebo be revealed.

For example, in a trial of hormone replacement therapy (HRT), there may be a placebo group plus three treatment groups (groups A, B, C and D) where each treatment group gets a different dose. Each patient in the trial gets identical-looking pills to take and the same directions, so neither they nor their trial doctor or nurse will know whether they are receiving a placebo or the HRT.

Thus randomisation and blinding prevent anyone involved in the clinical trial, including patients, from influencing – consciously or unconsciously – patient assignment to a clinical trial group. This is critically important because:

- The differences in patient characteristics between the test groups can affect the results more than the treatment itself if proper randomisation methods are not used;
- Any bias in the patient assignment process might yield misleading results about who the trial intervention works best in. Bias in the patient assignment process is sometimes referred to as *patient selection bias*. This is discussed in Text Box 4.2, which looks at how patient assignment might be carried out other than by randomisation; and/or
- Any bias in reporting the effects of the treatment may also yield misleading results. For example if patients know that they are taking a new treatment that they are very hopeful will benefit them, their hope may influence how they report feeling while on the treatment. Similarly, if a doctor knows that his or her patient is taking a treatment that he or she has spent a lot of time researching, it might affect how the doctor judges the patient's response to the treatment.

Text Box 4.2: Ways other than randomisation to assign patients to clinical trial groups

There are other ways that assignment to treatment groups could be done. For example the clinical trials team might choose to give the trial intervention to the trial participants:

- *They think could benefit the most* and standard treatment to others. Whilst this sounds logical, there are problems with this approach because at this point, the clinical trials team simply does not know how well the treatment works or in whom it works best. Taking this approach is really based on guessing rather than evidence; or
- *On a first-come-first-served basis.* For example, a trial opens for enrolment and the first 100 people with a particular medical condition who come in and enrol are given the experimental treatment. The next 100 people with the same condition who enrol are given the standard treatment. The results of the treatments given to the groups are compared. Is the comparison valid? Not really. There could be some differences between groups that were not accounted for. For instance, the first 100 people might have been more eager to receive the treatment, perhaps because they are the sickest, so they enrolled first and so the groups might have different patient characteristics. These differences could affect the trial's results independently from the effectiveness of the treatment itself. Results from the first group of patients might seem worse than results from the second group simply because the first group was sicker at the outset, not because the experimental treatment did not work.

Randomisation and *blinding* ensure that the clinical trial team gets as accurate a picture as possible – unbiased by the selection of patients – of the benefits and risks of the trial intervention.

In an emergency situation the clinical trial team can identify what group a patient is in. For example it was recently discovered that a commonly used drug increased the risk of cardiovascular disease in certain patients. The drug, Vioxx, was also being tested in a large worldwide clinical trial called VICTOR for a disease it had not been used for before. Vioxx was withdrawn from the market and the clinical trial team was given the confidential computer code to reveal patient assignments in the trial groups. Patients receiving Vioxx were notified immediately so that they could stop taking the medication and be checked for any side effects.

Understanding controls and placebos

A control group is used to allow comparison between the test intervention and:
- *The current standard diagnostic or treatment used at the time by the NHS*. The National Institute for Clinical Excellence (NICE) produces guidelines on what

drugs, surgical techniques or devices should be used for particular diseases. The guidelines are based on historical use and clinical trial evidence and determine what is considered current standard treatment. Standard treatments and diagnostics are those used first for patients with disease; it does not indicate how effective the treatment will be. For example, the standard treatment for the most common form of bacterial meningitis is very effective if given early; however, if the infection is not diagnosed early, other treatments may need to be used.

• *An 'inactive' form of the treatment or placebo.* A placebo is inactive. It is often designed to look exactly like the real treatment. Although a placebo is often thought of as a pill – which it may be for a drug trial – it can also be an injection, a physical manipulation, a device that is inactive or whatever harmless procedure is deemed an appropriate placebo for the trial. The important thing is that the placebo has the same appearance as the real treatment. A placebo is given only in trials in which the patient will not suffer any serious or long-term harm from receiving the placebo or sham (simulated device) treatment instead of active treatment. Thus, placebos are not used in trials in which patients have a life-threatening illness.

A control group consists of patients with similar characteristics who get an intervention other than the test intervention. A control can also mean giving the same patients different treatments at different points in the trial to compare their responses to the different treatments. Decisions about whether or what type of control is used are based on the International Conference on Harmonisation guidance on Good Clinical Practice (ICH-GCP) and on ethical principles and guidelines in human research (the Declaration of Helsinki, the Nuremberg Code and the Belmont Report). Then researchers use scientific principles about how to design a trial so it can yield the data they need to answer questions about safety and efficacy. The impact of proposed control groups on patient welfare is also considered by the research ethics committee reviewing the protocol. For example, placebo-controlled trials are considered unethical if effective, life-saving or life-prolonging treatment is available. Such trials are also unethical if patients assigned to a placebo group would likely suffer serious harm compared to those receiving an experimental treatment. Further information on regulations can be found in Chapter 5.

It is critically important to note that patients who receive a control – whether a standard intervention or a placebo – receive the same attention and follow-up as patients receiving the experimental treatment. The health of all patients in a clinical trial is carefully monitored by the doctors of the clinical trial team. If a patient's condition worsens significantly, the doctor may take the patient out of the trial and find out what treatment group the patient was in. If it was the placebo group, active treatment may be given. However, for many trials conducted in critically ill patients for whom there is no effective treatment, patients are usually not switched from one group to another. It is important to remember that placebos are not used in situations where the patient would be harmed by not receiving active treatment for the duration of the trial.

Why are placebos used in clinical trials?

If, by definition, a placebo is not treatment, why give it? Why not simply do nothing and compare that to the treatment group? The reason placebos are better than nothing is because of the *placebo effect*. For years, clinical trial teams have repeatedly observed that patients given a placebo often improve because of psychological effects rather than because of treatment effects. In other words, a treatment may have two effects: a psychological effect and a physical effect. Both may benefit the patient. For example, in clinical trials of anti-depressants it is common for patients receiving the placebo to improve significantly, even though they are not receiving the active treatment.

Patients may believe they are better simply because they believe they are receiving effective treatment. To determine whether the treatment is effective, the clinical trial team needs to subtract the impact of the placebo effect. When the control group is given a placebo (and the close medical monitoring that is part of the clinical trial), the placebo effect can be subtracted when the results of the experimental and control groups of the clinical trial are compared.

In some clinical trials, the clinical trial team may want to compare the effects of the medical intervention and placebo in the same patient. Patients will *cross over* from the test intervention to a placebo at particular times during the trial determined by randomisation. If it is a blinded crossover trial, the patient and the clinical trial team will not know which intervention the patient is receiving at a given time. A crossover trial design is normally used when a patient's disease is stable. The main benefits of a crossover trial are to:
- Reduce the number of patients needed in a study;
- Reduce the potential for results to be due to differences between patients.
- Assess whether the disease varies over time.

Patients will always be informed if a placebo is being used in a trial during the process in which they consent to take part in a clinical trial. (The process and issues of consent are covered in Chapter 3). However, if the clinical trial is a randomised placebo-controlled trial, it almost certainly will be *blinded* so that patients will not know which group they are in and whether they are receiving the placebo. The placebo effect can be significant and unpredictable. Whenever possible, patients are not told what treatment they are being given until the clinical trial is over. In this way, there is less chance that bias will be introduced from patients knowing which treatment they got. In fact, in many cases, the clinical trial is designed so that the researchers themselves will not know which patients are in the experimental or control groups. This helps reduce possible biases that could affect results.

What about trials that are not controlled or blinded?

Many trials are not controlled or blinded and are still very valid trials. Each clinical trial is designed to answer particular questions, and those questions differ for each trial. Depending on what the new treatment is, and depending on the stage of investigation, different types of trials are available for participation. Although the randomised controlled trial in which both the clinical trial team and the patients are blinded is the gold standard in clinical research, this type of trial may not always be possible or even preferable. For example, clinical trials:

- May be gathering preliminary data to see if a treatment is safe enough to warrant a full-scale trial and may have no control group;
- May be examining a treatment for a serious condition that has no alternative treatment, and randomisation would be unethical. In cases like these, the particular question the trial is designed to answer may preclude using randomisation or a control group. Trials like these might instead compare the results of the experimental treatment with the results of past trials that used a different treatment for the same condition;
- May have no need to use randomisation because patients serve as their own controls. For example, a trial may be trying to determine the best way to administer a particular treatment for a condition that varies greatly among patients. Individual diabetic patients, for example, can have very different responses to drugs that regulate their blood sugar levels. Each patient may be given two (or more) different drug regimens during the trial, so comparisons can be made within each patient; and
- May be unable to create a sham or look-alike treatment for a device or surgical procedure. Indeed it may be awkward or unethical to give a sham treatment. Also, the effects of treatment using a device might be apparent to the patient—such as use of an electrical stimulation device that creates a certain sensation that cannot be duplicated in sham treatment. In any event, participation in a trial should be tailored to provide the maximum protection to patients as well as to gather the maximum amount of useful data from the trial.

Understanding clinical trial results

The outcomes or endpoints clearly stated in a clinical trial protocol will form the basis of the results of the clinical trial. The assessment of survival will focus on how a patient responds to the treatment. Different responses in cancer trials, for example, include:

- *Complete response* – where the disease can no longer be detected for at least 4 weeks. A complete response is clearly a good indicator; however, it does not mean the disease is cured;
- *Partial response* – where the disease has improved for at least 4 weeks. For example in cancer a partial response is when the tumour decreases in size by at least half for at least 4 weeks and does not appear anywhere else in the body;

- *Progression* – where the disease gets worse by a set amount. Each disease has a different set of measurements that are used to determine when a disease has progressed; and
- *Stable disease* – where the disease does not progress or respond to treatment, but stays the same.

The length of time that the intervention has an effect on the patient's disease is important in understanding whether the intervention is worth the risks it may have or whether it is better than other available treatments. The *duration of response* is determined by the time between when the treatment was given and a response seen and any recurrence of disease. The *time to progression* is the length of time between starting the intervention and the disease progressing.

Summary

To make well-informed decisions about whether or not to enter a clinical trial, a patient needs to understand clinical trial jargon. The words and phrases outlined in this chapter describe important concepts in clinical trials, such as whether a patient will receive an active or inactive intervention; whether a patient will know what he or she is receiving; and what the results of the trial mean.

The main concepts that need to be fully explained and understood include:
- *Randomisation*, which explains the random assignment of patients to different groups in a trial. Randomisation is usually done by a computer and aims to reduce the chance of other factors, not being analysed in the trial, affecting the result. Randomisation helps to ensure that the results of the trial give clear answers about the intervention being tested;
- *Controlled trials*, where one group of patients does not receive the test intervention. The control group will often receive the current standard treatment for their disease or they may receive a placebo. This allows for comparison of the test intervention with the standard treatment and reduces effects caused by other factors;
- A *placebo* is a type of control that looks the same and is taken in the same way as the test intervention, but is inactive. The purpose of the placebo is so that factors other than the effects of the test intervention itself can be calculated and taken into account when analysing trial results;
- *Blinding* is a technique that is used to reduce bias in clinical trials. Blinding can take two forms:
  - Single blinding – to reduce patient bias by not telling a patient whether he or she is in the test intervention or the control group; and
  - Double blinding – to reduce patient and doctor bias by not telling either patients or healthcare professionals whether the patients are receiving the test intervention or the control treatment.

- Patients' *response* to treatment is a measurement of how much their disease responds to the medical intervention. A response is measured in terms of disease improvement over time, and is measured differently for different diseases. A positive response can be complete or partial and a negative response is called progression. If the disease is stable it means that the disease has stayed the same, not progressed or responded to treatment.

CHAPTER 5

Questions About Clinical Trials: A Framework for Discussion

Research has found that some people participating in clinical trials tend to do better than similar patients receiving standard diagnostic or treatment intervention outside of trials. However, participation in a clinical trial is entirely voluntary. Therefore, a patient must give his or her permission, or consent, to be entered into a clinical trial. A patient's decision to decline taking part in a clinical trial will be respected, and will not affect the quality of the patient's medical care in any way. Information, for example, about why other people have chosen to take part or not take part in a clinical trial, will help patients weigh up the benefits and risks of a clinical trial. How an individual patient measures benefit and risk is an important and very personal decision.

This chapter of the guide provides a framework within which patients and their healthcare professionals can consider together the issues known to be important in informing this decision-making process. It is written in a question-and-answer format covering the following issues:

- *What are patient's rights?* – This section looks at the need for patients to give permission to take part in a trial, a patient's right to withdraw at any time and patient confidentiality;
- *Why do patients take part in clinical trials?* This section looks at quality of care and clinical outcomes associated with trial participation, together with research on key motivations for taking part in clinical trials;
- *Why do patients decline to take part?* – This section looks at motivations for declining to take part in a clinical trial, together with why patients might choose to withdraw from a trial;
- *What empowers patients?* – This section looks at how patients can ensure their own safety, whom patients can talk to, including other patients and what to do if something goes wrong;
- *What are the implications of taking part in a trial?* – This section looks at implications in terms of extra support from carers and the potential for any financial burdens.

What are patient's rights?

Can a patient withdraw from a clinical trial at any time?

Yes. A patient is free to withdraw from the clinical trial at any time, without giving a reason. No one should try to persuade patients to continue to participate if they do not want to. Again, a patient's decision to withdraw from a trial will not affect the patient's quality of medical care in any way. However, if the patient is having a new treatment as part of the trial, he or she may not be able to continue having the treatment but will be given the appropriate available standard treatment. Once withdrawn, patients may still wish, and have the opportunity, to participate in follow-up visits. The clinical trial team will usually want to follow up with patients who have left the trial after receiving even partial treatment. Even patients who withdraw provide important information to the trial.

Will the confidentiality of patient's medical records be respected?

Yes. In the age of the information superhighway, many people have become aware of issues about privacy, especially regarding health matters and who can access medical records. Some of the reasons for concern include fear of stigmatisation because of a serious illness and possible employment or insurance discrimination.

A patient's medical records concerning the clinical trial remain confidential. No one who looks at the notes can give information to anyone outside the clinical trial team looking after the patient. Within clinical trials, participant names are 'masked' and patients are identified in records by a numbering system so that anyone looking at individual patient information sees a code rather than a name. Officials from organisations that sponsor or fund trials may inspect and copy clinical records to verify information submitted by a sponsor. This is normally done only if a legal issue arises, and always has the patient's personal details removed so that they cannot be identified. Consent forms should clearly explain that when a patient participates in research, the patient's records automatically become part of the research database. Patients do not have the option to keep their records from being audited or reviewed by organisations with trial oversight including the Medicines and Healthcare Products Regulatory Authority (MHRA). When an individually identifiable medical record (usually kept by the clinical researcher) is copied and reviewed by an oversight organisation, proper confidentiality procedures are followed to protect patient privacy.

In the same way, when the results of the trial are published, the patients involved will not be identified. It is important to note that trial participants are not identified personally in published articles; articles that report individual patient data typically refer to individuals by a letter or number. Information about the sex and age of participants and medical characteristics is often included, but nothing identifies an individual.

If something goes wrong, will the patient receive compensation?

Yes. The diagnostic tests and treatments used in clinical trials conform to the highest standards. Commercial organisations manufacturing the diagnostics or treatments are insured so that if a patient is damaged by some unforeseen event, compensation can be paid. It is rare for patients to be harmed in this way, although in some drug trials the trial participants may suffer unpleasant side effects.

Clinical trials funded by the Department of Health or the UK Medical Research Council may not have this kind of insurance, but a payment would be made if something did go wrong. Individual NHS Trusts are responsible for insuring themselves against damage caused by local studies, and research ethics committees would refuse approval for trials where there is no insurance.

All compensation agreements involving the pharmaceutical industry follow the guidelines of the Association of British Pharmaceutical Industry (ABPI).

Why do patients take part in clinical trials?

Do patients who enter clinical trials do better than those who do not?

Some research has found that some people participating in clinical trials tend to do better than similar patients outside trials, receiving standard diagnostic or treatment intervention.

For example, ECRI conducted a systematic review that found that cancer and heart disease patients treated in phase II or phase III trials survive longer than patients who are not treated in trials. ECRI researchers analysed four published studies on cancer patients and one published study of heart disease patients that compared the treatment outcomes of patients in phase II and III trials to outcomes of patients who were eligible for those trials but did not participate. (Patients treated outside the trials did not necessarily receive the same treatment as patients in the trials.)

Four studies found that cancer patients in clinical trials survived significantly longer than patients who were eligible for, but did not participate in, the trials. In the study on heart disease patients, a survival difference in the direction of improvement over patients not in the trial was seen, but this difference was not statistically significant. Further details of this research can be found in Appendix B.

Thus, there is some evidence that patients in phase II or phase III trials survive longer than similar patients who are not in trials. This apparent advantage may be due to better treatment, better patient monitoring by healthcare professionals or other factors. However, since there were only five studies available for analysis, it cannot be concluded that these results apply to all patients inside and outside trials. Larger studies that control adequately for various important patient characteristics are necessary to confirm these results.

What kind of care can be expected in a clinical trial?

Clinical trials are carefully designed to minimise the risks and maximise the benefits to all patients who take part, regardless of whether they are randomised to the trial group receiving the new intervention or to the control group receiving the standard intervention or a placebo. Chapter 4 provides details on randomisation to trial and control groups.

Patients can expect to receive excellent medical care for their condition in a clinical trial. Typically, patients in clinical trials are more closely monitored during and after the trial than patients treated outside clinical trials. This is because the trial protocol requires detailed collection of data and frequent patient check-ups to assess how patients are doing. This means a patient in a clinical trial will have regular tests, often more than to those received during standard care. Patients are also usually asked extra questions about how they are feeling; sometimes patients are asked to fill in questionnaires or keep a diary.

In addition, the clinical trial doctors and nurses typically come from among the clinicians who are most knowledgeable about the disease or condition under study – it is the focus of their work. The sponsors and other funding agencies also have high standards that must be met. These organisations usually inspect clinical trial sites to make sure that the standards of the clinical trial can be met, especially with regard to patient care and safety.

The benefit to the patient of this extra attention is that any changes in his or her health – whether or not they are related to the clinical trial – are frequently picked up and acted upon earlier than for patients receiving standard care. However, all this means that patients may need to go to the hospital or to see their general practitioner (GP) more frequently than normal. Therefore, it may be more tiring for the patient and may cost more money for travel.

Why do patients decide to take part in clinical trials?

In ECRI's analysis of why patients participate in trials, the three most commonly cited reasons that patients gave for participating in a clinical trials were:
- Hope of some personal therapeutic benefit, reported by 16–100% of patients in different trials;
- Confidence in their doctor's recommendation to enter a trial, reported by 0–63% of patients in different trials; and
- Hope of benefiting others, reported by 0–65% of patients in different trials.

ECRI used statistical methods to try to estimate the typical percentage of patients who cited these reasons over all the studies. ECRI found that an estimated 45% of patients cited personal benefit, 30% of patients cited doctor influence and 21% of patients cited a desire to benefit others. Other reasons for participating cited by patients varied widely. They included:
- No other alternative
- Family/friend influence
- Better to do something than having no treatment
- Better monitoring of condition
- Pressured to enrol by clinical trial personnel

- Nothing to lose
- Have the time to do it
- Trust in institution, doctors, nurses
- Don't know why, just did it.

Further details of this research can be found in Appendix B.

Why do patients decline to take part in a clinical trial or withdraw from a clinical trial they are involved in?

Why do patients decline to take part in clinical trials?

A patient's decision to decline taking part in a clinical trial will be respected. The decision not to take part will not affect the patient's quality of medical care in any way. Whilst the patient does not need to give an explanation of his or her decision, the most common reasons cited for not participating in clinical trials are:

- Fear of being allocated or randomised to the control group of the trial, i.e. that group of the trial which receives an inactive form of the new treatment or the standard of care. This reason was reported by 1–31% of patients who declined trial participation;
- Too far to travel was reported by 11–37% of patients; and
- Desire to have the doctor choose the treatment rather than accept a process that uses randomisation to assign patients to a treatment group was reported by 0–18% of patients.

Notice that the percentage did not exceed 37% for any one reason. When ECRI used statistical methods to estimate the prevalence of reasons given for not participating in a trial, the highest percentage was for travel concerns (23%) and the lowest percentage was for the desire to have the doctor choose the treatment (11%). Other reasons given for not participating (in no particular order of frequency) were:

- Preference for receiving standard treatment
- Fear or dislike being treated like a 'guinea pig'
- Lack of insurance coverage for clinical trials
- Complex consent process
- Unable to give consent
- Doctor objected
- Family objected
- Not interested
- Condition deteriorating
- Inconvenient
- Dislike focusing on disease
- Not enough time

Why do patients withdraw from a clinical trial?

Whilst a patient withdrawing from a clinical trial is not obliged to give a reason, the clinical trial team will want to understand his or her reasons. It is important for the clinical trial team to know why a patient has withdrawn so they can account for what happened to all patients involved and assess the effects of the intervention on all patients enrolled. Patients withdraw from a clinical trial for a number of reasons, the most common reasons include:

- *Fear of being randomised to the control group* – even though the main purpose of a clinical trial is to advance medical knowledge in a way that will benefit future patients, the main reason most people enter a trial is the hope that they may improve their health. This is a perfectly valid reason for participating in a clinical trial. In a blinded trial, patients may come to think that they have been randomised to the control group receiving standard treatment or to the placebo group receiving an inactive form of the treatment, and therefore choose to withdraw. They may think this because of the way they are feeling, by comparing notes with other patients or by information gained from talking to members of the clinical trial team. In an unblinded trial, the patients know if they have been assigned to the control or placebo group, and can therefore choose to withdraw on the basis of this information. Whilst this is understandable, it is important to remember that evidence suggests that patients in clinical trials fare better on the whole than similar patients who receive treatment outside a trial. It is important to discuss this aspect of clinical trial participation before a patient consents to enter a trial;
- *Side effects* – patients may withdraw from clinical trials because they experience side effects that they are unable to tolerate. This is usually more common in early-phase trials of new interventions. It is particularly important that patients who withdraw from a trial for this reason report the side effects whilst in the trial and when they withdraw. It is important for the clinical trial team to collect important safety and efficacy information. This will help reduce the risk to other clinical trial participants.

How can patients be empowered during their involvement in a clinical trial?

How can patients ensure their own safety?

Each patient is his or her own best protection against harm. Patients can do this by:

- *Fully disclosing to the trial doctor and research nurse medical history, current state of health and medication.* It is important that patients make sure that their medical records are available to the trial doctors. Patients should confirm that the research doctor and their other doctors are communicating about what is happening during the clinical trial and outside the trial in terms of any care received. This includes even the most seemingly insignificant event, e.g. patients should let their doctors know that they are taking a vitamin C supplement to help a cold. It is the patient's responsibility to be as honest and open as possible about any changes he or she makes for health, and the doctor's responsibility to respect the patient's decisions and take all things into consideration. For patients on a trial, it is very important to promptly report any side effects to the clinical trial team, even if they are not sure that the symptoms or side effects are related to the treatment;

- *Fully disclosing to the designated person, usually the trial doctor or nurse, anything the patient did that he/she was not supposed to do.* This is called doing something that is 'off-protocol'. If this happens, for example if a treatment is missed, the patient should quickly contact the person designated on the consent form. It is not possible in advance to know what the consequences of doing something off-protocol would be, but it is very important that the clinical trial team know about it as soon as possible to help ensure patient health and safety. Off-protocol events should be recorded in as much detail as possible. Mistakes happen, and a patient's ability to comply with the treatment is a valuable part of the information collected during a trial. Clinical trials not only find out how well a new treatment works, they also find out how easy or difficult it is for patients to follow the treatment regimen. If many patients have the same difficulty, the clinical trial team may realise that they need to revise some aspect of treatment or instructions about how to follow the regimen. Thus, it is important that patients and the clinical trial team can speak openly and honestly about this issue.

Who can patients talk to?

Patient information sheets, available for every trial, are a good source of information on who to contact and often provide answers to common questions. Information is also provided on who can be contacted:

- If something goes wrong – when a patient joins a trial, he or she will be given the name and contact details of a member of the clinical trial team who can be contacted 24 hours a day if a serious side effect or complication arises;
- The clinical trial doctor or nurse provides the first point of contact for patients seeking information on participating in a clinical trial and helps with non-emergency queries or concerns about care during a trial, for example, by discussing the possible side effects of treatment;
- The clinical trial management team can answer queries about the trial, particularly if patient safety is of concern, when they should be notified. The clinical trial management team can also refer the patient and carer to the appropriate member of the clinical trial team;
- A patient advocate for the trial, if one is available, can provide the patient perspective;
- A patient advisor from the ethics committee, if there is one, may be available to discuss queries or concerns about ethical aspects of the trial.

Can patients involved in clinical trials share their experience with other participating patients?

Patients who have participated in clinical trials often say they feel supported and comforted by being part of a group of patients with the same disease or condition. It is natural and useful that patients exchange views on their experiences during the trial.

However, discussing certain things about the trial may not be helpful. For example, if patients in the trial discuss their response to the trial intervention to try and work out whether they are in the trial group or the control group. People often respond very differently to the same intervention, so comparing notes with other patients on the trial is unlikely to uncover which group a patient is in.

What can patients do in the event of an emergency or serious side effect?

Ultimately, the clinical trial team is responsible for dealing with side effects and complications. Practically speaking, the location for receiving treatment depends on where the patient is when a side effect or complication occurs:

- *If the side effect or complication is serious* – the patient, with the help of a family member or friend, should seek care at the nearest available hospital or GP practice and should let the treating doctors know whom to contact in the trial. The treating doctors will need vital medical information from the clinical trial team about the treatment so that the necessary consultations can take place to treat the complication or side effect appropriately. The consent form should explicitly state who is responsible for treating unexpected side effects.
- *If the side effect does not require urgent attention and the patient has time* – the patient should contact and visit his or her clinical trial doctor or research nurse.

What can a patient do if his or her condition deteriorates during a clinical trial?

Each patient, his or her health professional and clinical trial team should discuss what action to take if the patient's condition worsens. Unfortunately, the worsening of a patient's condition is not an unusual event if the patient has a life-threatening condition and the disease has progressed. The clinical trial doctors closely monitor each patient to observe the effects of treatment during the trial to see how well it is working. If the treatment itself is believed to be causing unexpected deterioration, the clinical trial doctors will do everything possible to halt or reverse that effect – including withdrawing the patient from the trial. Again, patients can withdraw at any time should they feel unable to continue on the trial.

What can a patient do if the treatment has an unexpected effect?

Some uncertainty and risk are always part of clinical research. Similarly, uncertainty is often part of the picture in standard medical practice. Unfortunately, no one, not even the clinical trial team who designed the trial, knows all the possible side effects or complications. The very reasons for doing medical research are to detect the risks as well as the benefits of treatment. Unexpected complications and side effects can happen, especially in early-phase trials, when the basic safety and efficacy data are just being collected. The more people on whom a new treatment is tested, the more we learn about side effects and how often they occur. Detecting rare side effects requires studying a lot of people – 1000 or more – simply to detect the effect. Long-term safety is not really known for any treatment until that treatment has been used for a while on a large number of patients.

Will patients involved in clinical trials need extra help and support from their carers?

It is important for patients and healthcare professionals to consider the impact of participation in the clinical trial on the need of the patient for extra help from their carers during the trial. Will patients have the social support system needed to help during the trial? Having a good support system in place outside the trial can affect how well patients feel emotionally, how well they can comply with the trial protocol and whether they complete the trial. Depending on the trial being considering, additional support from family and friends may be needed, e.g. running errands; providing transportation for errands and clinical trial treatment and check-ups; shopping, cooking, or cleaning; caring for other family members, such as children or elders; or caring for pets. Patients may also need more emotional and moral support from family and friends at different times during the trial if the treatment is difficult to tolerate.

What are the likely costs of and reimbursement for patients participating in clinical trials?

In the UK, we are lucky to have free access to healthcare through the NHS. So the cost implications of a clinical trial are the more indirect and intangible costs:

- *Indirect costs* that patients might incur include the costs for travel, accommodation and additional lost time from work when participating in a trial and also for carers who accompany them. The clinical trial research coordinator may be able to help determine what those costs for a patient would amount to over the full course of the trial. They may also have resources for accommodation to be provided for patients participating in a trial and their carers. In studies analysed by ECRI, the need to travel to participate in a trial was the most common reason patients gave for not participating
- *Intangible costs* include those such as separation from carers during the trial and other quality-of-life issues in terms of how the trial affects a patient's activities of daily living. For example, side effects from treatment, even if they are deemed 'minor' and 'temporary', such as nausea, can significantly affect a patient's activities and feelings.

Therefore, it is important that healthcare professionals and patients consider the potential impact of the trial on their activities, quality of life and relationships with carers. All patients enrolling in a trial must be informed of any costs they may incur and the potential for reimbursement.

There are some trials that pay participants for their involvement. Payment of this type is usually for studies involving healthy volunteers and is not considered a benefit. It is thought of as a recruitment incentive. Financial incentives are often used when health benefits to subjects are remote or non-existent in the trial. All information about payment, including the amount and schedule of payment(s), must be included in the consent document, following approval from the ethics committee.

Summary

Understandably, patients will often have many questions when considering clinical trial participation. This chapter addresses a number of the most common questions, and aims to help both patients and their doctors openly discuss:

What a patient's rights are: The most common questions about patients' rights are around:

- *Informed consent* – the final decision on whether to take part in a clinical trial must be the patient's. When a patient chooses to give consent to participate the trial team must ensure that the patient has received and understood as much information on the trial as he or she needs;
- *Withdrawal from a trial* – it is each patient's right to withdraw from the trial at any point in time, without reason;
- *Confidentiality* – medical records for patients in a clinical trial must be kept confidential; and
- *What happens if something goes wrong* – in the UK the organisations involved in clinical trials are covered by insurance. Therefore if something unexpected goes wrong the patient will be able to seek compensation. This will be awarded after the appropriate legal process has been completed.

The reasons patients give for choosing to take part in clinical trials: Patients choose to take part in clinical trials because:

- There is some evidence that patients in clinical trials do better than those treated outside a trial and the doctors who run clinical trials are usually experts in the patient's disease;
- There is hope that a new treatment may be beneficial, particularly when a patient has not responded to any other available treatments;
- They are confident that the recommendations made by their doctor is in their best interest; and
- They hope that their participation will benefit future patients.

The reasons patients give for declining to take part in a clinical trial: Patients choose to decline taking part in clinical trials because:

- They do not want to be randomised to a group that may receive an inactive treatment or standard treatment;

- It is too far to travel and the demands on their time are too great. This is a part of the impact of the trial on a patient's quality of life;
- They would rather that their doctor choose their treatment, rather than be randomly assigned one.

How patients can be empowered: Understanding of good quality information can empower patients to:

- Ensure that they are safe by being aware of the potential for harm and disclosing all medical information;
- Talk to the right people about challenges they may be facing or questions they have. This is most often a member of the clinical trial team;
- Share experiences with other trial participants – many patients say that they feel comforted knowing that they can talk to people in the same situation as them; and
- Know what to do in an emergency situation, if their condition deteriorates or if a patient experiences an unexpected effect.

What the potential implications of taking part in a clinical trial are: It is important that patients fully understand the expectations a clinical trial places on them, including:

- *Extra support from carers* – who may need to help with things like shopping and transport
- *The costs to a patient* – including financial costs such as travel and accommodation. In some trials these costs may be reimbursed and impact on quality of life.

Finding Out About Clinical Trials that are Currently or Soon to be Recruiting

A number of organisations give information about clinical trials and where they are being carried out. The website addresses for some of these are given in the table below. Although a few of these are based in the US, they sometimes list clinical trials in the UK and Europe.

General

Medical Research Council Clinical Trials	www.ctu.mrc.ac.uk
Current Controlled Trials	www.controlled-trials.com
National Institutes of Health (NIH)	http://www.clinicaltrials.gov
National Research Register	http://www.nrr.nhs.uk/
Involve	http://www.invo.org.uk/Database.asp
National Electronic Library for Health	http://www.nelh.nhs.uk/clinicaltrials/

For Specific Diseases

Cancer Research UK	www.cancerhelp.org.uk/trials
National Cancer Research Network	www.ncrn.org.uk/portfoliodbase
Cancer Guide	www.cancerguide.org
National Translational Cancer Research Network	www.ntrac.org.uk
Lung Research	www.researchvolunteers.co.uk
Royal Marsden Hospital	www.royalmarsden.org
Breakthrough Breast Cancer	www.breakthrough.org.uk
Leukemia Research	www.lrf.org.uk
Centre Watch	www.centerwatch.com/cwworld
National AIDS Manual	http://www.aidsmap.com/en/docs/ux/ treatment.asp

---

APPENDIX B: ECRI Evidence Report

Patients' Reasons for Participation in Clinical Trials and Effect of Trial Participation on Patient Outcomes

Policy Statement

This report is a short-form evidence report designed to provide a rapid and accurate overview of some aspects of patient behavior regarding clinical trials and a comparison of patient outcomes inside and outside of clinical trials. The information contained in this report derives from the currently available published, peer-reviewed scientific literature, and studies chosen for inclusion were limited to English-language publications. The recommendations and conclusions must be interpreted cautiously and judiciously. The data on which they are based often do not permit unequivocal resolution of the scientific and clinical issues most relevant to patient care. ECRI implies no warranty and assumes no liability for the information, conclusions, and recommendations in this evidence report.

ECRI believes that the sources of information used in this report are reliable and has used its best professional judgment in analyzing the data obtained, but cannot assume any liability for the accuracy or completeness of the studies undertaken by others. ECRI makes no recommendations about the applicability for an individual patient or the appropriateness of an individual insurance coverage decision. Such decisions are the responsibility of the patient, his or her physician, and the insurance carrier. This report should not be used to judge the economic value or marketplace dynamics associated with a technology for investment or other business purposes. There may be little relationship between the clinical value of a technology and the financial performance of companies associated with the technology.

The conclusions and recommendations of this report and the studies on which it is based are highly perishable and reflect the state of the art at the time this report was compiled. A multidisciplinary staff of life and physical scientists and health professionals produced this report. This report was carefully reviewed by other professionals within ECRI as well as by qualified extramural reviewers in pertinent fields before being issued as a final report. Neither ECRI nor its employees accept gifts, grants, or contributions from or consult for medical device or pharmaceutical manufacturers. This report reflects the judgment of ECRI and not necessarily those of outside reviewers.

The Health Technology Assessment Information Service (HTAIS) provides evidence reports and information about healthcare technology and services to support to help governments, hospitals, health systems, managed care organizations, health insurers, health professionals, and the public meet the challenge of evaluating healthcare technology objectively and rationally. HTAIS disseminates information derived from its assessments to consumers and patients to help inform their decision making about healthcare options.

HTAIS is a service of ECRI, a nonprofit health services research agency and a Collaborating Center for Healthcare Technology Assessment of the World Health Organization. ECRI has been designated an Evidence-based Practice Center by the U.S. Agency for Healthcare Research and Quality. ECRI's mission is to provide information and technical assistance to the healthcare community worldwide to support safe and cost-effective patient care. The results of ECRI's research and experience are available through its publications, information systems, databases, technical assistance programs, laboratory services, seminars, and fellowships.

ECRI
5200 Butler Pike
Plymouth Meeting, PA 19462
Telephone: (610) 825-6000   Fax: (610) 834-1275
http://www.ecri.org

Overview

Participation in Clinical Trials

This report is an evidence-based supplement to ECRI's *Patient Reference Guide for Adults with a Serious or Life-Threatening Illness: Should I Enter a Clinical Trial?* (Freely available online at ECRI's Web site "Patient Information" tab at www.ecri.org.) Patients may have several questions and concerns as they consider enrolling in a clinical trial. The patient reference guide is an educational resource that explains concepts and terms that may be unfamiliar to patients, such as the phases of trials, weighing risks and benefits of trial participation, randomization, placebo controls, and double-blinding. In addition, it contains practical resources designed to assist patients with the decision of whether to participate (such as a list of questions to ask a physician). Furthermore, the guide informs patients of key issues that affect patients entering trials, such as informed consent, patient protection mechanisms, and the right to withdraw from the trial at any time.

The patient reference guide refers to research relevant to the enrollment decision. This report contains a detailed summary and analysis of that research evidence on two particular questions:

1 *What reasons do patients give for participating and not participating in clinical trials?*
2 *Do patients in clinical trials have better treatment outcomes than similar patients who were not in clinical trials?*

These questions do not exhaust the set of evidence-based questions that are important to patients in the decision-making process. We selected them because in our judgment they are important questions, and because our literature searches uncovered evidence that bears directly on them.

An evidence-based approach is important because it does not rely the impressions or memories of individuals. Impressions and memory are imperfect and may be subject to the biases of a particular person. This report relies on information that has been systematically collected by researchers as part of an implicit effort to overcome these imperfections and possible biases. We therefore excluded information that is potentially biased. As such, the evidence upon which this report is based is derived not merely from studies that have been published in the medical literature, but from the highest-quality studies in that literature.

For clarity of terminology, in this report we have distinguished between a "study" and a "trial." Research articles that addressed the first question are referred to as "studies." For example, a "study" might report the reasons that patients cited for why they participated in any of three cancer trials. By contrast, research articles that addressed the second question are referred to as "trials." For example, a patient might enroll in a "trial" of a new chemotherapeutic drug for the treatment of cancer.

Evidence Base

Identification of Clinical Studies

One characteristic of a good evidence-based analysis is a systematic and comprehensive search for information. Such searches distinguish ECRI's assessments from traditional literature reviews. With a less rigorous approach to identifying and obtaining literature, it is possible for a reviewer to include only articles that agree with a particular perspective and to ignore articles that do not. Our approach precludes this potential reviewer bias because we obtained and included articles according to explicitly determined a priori criteria.

We excluded some articles that we obtained because of their relatively low methodological quality. This is because the results of these articles can be misleading. We document these exclusions in the "Study Selection" section of this report. Articles that we included are discussed in the "Results" section.

To identify information for this report, we searched the following databases:
Bioethicsline (through November 2001)
Cochrane Library (through 2001, Issue 3)
ECRI Library Catalog (through December 2001)
PubMed (includes Medline, PreMedline, and HealthSTAR) (1988 through
    November 2001)
U.K. National Health Service (NHS) Centre for Reviews and Dissemination
    Web site (through November 2001)
U.S. National Institutes of Health (NIH) Web site (through November 2001)
U.S. National Library of Medicine (NLM) LocatorPlus (through November
    2001)

The search strategies employed a number of freetext keywords as well as
controlled vocabulary terms including (but not limited to) the following concepts:

Main concept: Clinical trials

Additional concepts: altruism; altruistic; attitude; attitude to health; benefit; ben-
    eficial; conflict of interest; control group; cooperative behavior; decision-
    making; enlist; enroll; equipoise; ethics; financial disclosure; financial ties;
    finder's fees; fraud; join; Helsinki; human experimentation; informed con-
    sent; insider dealing; institutional review boards; IRB; medical errors;
    motivation; patient acceptance of healthcare; patient compliance; patient
    participation; patient satisfaction; patients; physician-patient relationships;
    placebo effect; random allocation; recruit; risk; social perception; social val-
    ues; survival; treatment outcome; truth disclosure; voluntary workers; vol-
    unteers; well-being

In addition, we hand-searched the following bibliography:
National Library of Medicine. Ethical issues in research involving human par-
    ticipants. National Library of Medicine. Bethesda (MD):1999; 296 p. (Cur-
    rent Bibliographies in Medicine; 99–3).
This resource contains 4,640 citations published between January 1989 and
    November 1998. It is available at *http://www.nlm.nih.gov/pubs/cbm/hum_exp
    .html*.

What reasons do patients give for participating and not participating in clinical trials?

The primary audience for the patient reference guide is patients who are considering whether to enroll in a clinical trial. We posed this question because
such patients may find it helpful to know the reasons that other patients give
for their decisions. We considered reasons *for* participation as well as reasons
against participation to provide a balanced analysis.

Study Selection

We selected studies based on predetermined objective criteria. We employed
these criteria to ensure that we selected articles in an unbiased manner. The

criteria that we used were specifically designed to include only those studies that were most likely to have valid conclusions and be most relevant to patients considering enrollment in a clinical trial. A research analyst evaluated study design and quality of reporting without reference to the specific results reported by the study. We required studies to meet the following four criteria for inclusion in our analysis:

- *Studies included mentally competent patients with an acute or chronic life-threatening illness.* Only studies of life-threatening illnesses were considered because the intended audience for the patient reference guide is patients with a life-threatening illness who are considering enrollment in clinical trials.
- *All patients were at least 18 years old.* Parents and caregivers make decisions for entering children into clinical trials, and the reasons for such proxy decision making may not be representative of reasons given by individual adult patients.
- *All patients had been asked to participate in an actual clinical trial.* Studies based on patients' hypothetical decision making were not included because patients' reasons for making hypothetical choices may not accurately reflect their reasons for real decisions.
- *Patients were asked to provide their own reason(s) for participating or not participating in a clinical trial.* We did not consider the opinions of physicians, caregivers, family members, or any other parties regarding patients' reasons for participation. Their opinions may be different from the reasons stated by patients themselves; for this report, we adopted a purely patient-oriented approach.

Seventeen studies met the above inclusion criteria. We excluded 3 of the 17 for reasons listed in **Table B.1**. These studies were qualitative and did not report numbers or percentages of patients who cited each reason.

The remaining 14 studies **(Table B.2)** reported information gathered from 2,189 patients who provided reasons for participating in a trial, and 6,498 patients who provided reasons against participating in a trial. Eleven studies reported reasons for trial participation, and four studies reported reasons against trial participation (one study reported reasons for and against participation). Six studies asked questions in an open-ended format (e.g., "Why did you

Table B.1 Excluded Studies

Study	Reason for exclusion
Huizinga et al.(2)	Did not report the number or percentage of patients who gave each reason
Schutta and Burnett(3)	Did not report the number or percentage of patients who gave each reason
Searight and Miller(4)	Did not report the number or percentage of patients who gave each reason

Table B.2 Study Characteristics

Author and year	Disease	n	Mean age	% female	Reasons for participation	Reasons against participation	Open-ended question	Closed-ended question	>1 reason per patient	Phase I
Taylor and Leitman (2001)(5)	Cancer	5,972	NR	NR		✓	✓		✓	NR
Jenkins and Fallowfield (2000)(6)	Cancer	185[a]	NR	69.6%[b]	✓	✓	✓	✓		
Ling et al. (2000)(7)	Cancer	163	60[b,c]	65%[b]		✓	✓	✓		Mix
Tomamichel et al. (2000)(8)	Cancer	31	57[c]	29%	✓			✓		✓
Yuval et al. (2000)(9)	MI	150	NR	NR	✓			✓		✓
Hutchison (1998)(1)	Cancer	28	55.4	39.3%	✓			✓		✓
Itoh et al. (1997)(10)	Cancer	32	58[c]	53.1%	✓			✓	✓	✓
Daugherty et al. (1995)(11)	Cancer	27	58[c]	29.6%	✓		✓	✓	✓	✓
Henzlova et al. (1994)(12)	LVD	1,162	NR	NR	✓			✓	✓	
Wilcox and Schroer (1994)(13)	Heart disease	40	65.8	45%	✓		✓		✓	
Smith and Arnesen (1988)(14)	MI	178	64[b]	31%[b]		✓		✓	✓	
Mattson et al. (1985)(15)	MI	380	54[b]	NR	✓		✓			
Penman et al. (1984)(16)	Cancer	144	NR	52%	✓			✓		
Rodenhuis et al. (1984)(17)	Cancer	10	NR	40%	✓		✓		✓	✓
Totals	Cancer: 9 Heart: 5	3502	59	45%	13*	4	6	9	7	5

a—Jenkins and Fallowfield(6) reported 138 patients who gave reasons for participation and 47 patients who gave reasons against participation

b—Based on the total number of patients in the study, not the number of patients for whom reasons were reported

c—Median age

Mix—Ling et al.(7) included 19 trials: two were phase I, nine were phase II or later, and for eight, study phase could not be determined

n—Number of patients for whom reasons were reported

LVD—Left ventricular dysfunction; MI—Myocardial infarction; NR—Not reported decide to participate?"), and nine studies asked questions in a closed-ended format (e.g., "Among the reasons listed below, select the one that describes why you decided to participate"). One study used both open- and closed-ended questions.

Seven studies permitted patients to list more than one reason, but only one of these (Hutchison(1)) asked patients to rank-order their reasons. In the remaining six studies, patients were not asked about the relative importance of the listed reasons. Five studies addressed participation in phase I trials, and seven studies addressed participation in phase II or phase III trials (one did not report trial phase(s), and another contained a mix of phase I and non-phase I trials).

Key Study Results

The included studies reported several different kinds of results, but not all of these results were directly relevant to the question. Therefore, we only considered the relevant subset of results. These results were comprised of: (1) a set of reasons cited by patients for or against participation, and (2) for each reason, the percentage of patients who cited that reason.

Results

Reasons for participation

Table B.3 shows each reason for participating in a clinical trial and the percentage of patients who reported it. Studies often used different verbal descriptions of the same general reason category. For example, Jenkins and Fallowfield(6) found that 16.3% of patients gave the reason "I thought the trial/study offered the best treatment available," whereas Tomamichel et al.(8) reported that 59% of patients participated because of the "possibility of medical benefit." Both of these reasons can be assigned to the general category "potential health benefit." In order to compare the results of different studies, ECRI assigned each specific reason to one of three general categories: potential health benefit, physician influence, and potential benefit to others (i.e., altruism). Another ECRI research analyst independently checked these assignments, and all disagreements were resolved by discussion. The category assignments appear in the rightmost column of **Table B.3**.

Some studies reported more than one reason within a single general category. For example, Yuval et al.(9) found that 31% of patients gave the reason "Hoped for better treatment" and 12% of patients gave the reason "Hoped for better follow-up." ECRI assigned both of these reasons to the general category "potential health benefit." We added the two percentages to yield 43% as the percentage of patients in the Yuval et al. study who gave a reason within the general category of potential health benefit. We performed similar computations in other studies where appropriate.

Table B.3 Reasons for Participation

Author	n	Reported reasons for participation	Percent of patients[a]	Reason category assigned by ECRI
Jenkins and Fallowfield(6)	147	I feel that others with my illness will benefit from the results of the trial	23.1%	Potential benefit to others
		I trusted the doctor treating me	21.1%	Physician influence
		I thought the trial/study offered the best treatment available	16.3%	Potential health benefit
		Other	41.5%	Other
Tomamichel et al.(8)	31	Possibility of medical benefit	59%	Potential health benefit
		Trust in institutional oncologist	26%	Physician influence
		Contribution to research	3%	Potential benefit to others
		Other	12%	Other
Yuval et al.(9)	150	To help research	35%	Potential benefit to others
		Hoped for better treatment	31%	Potential health benefit
		Don't know	14%	Other
		Hoped for better follow-up	12%	Potential health benefit
		Was frightened to refuse	8%	Other
Hutchison(1)	28	Might help you	Median rank 1[b]	Potential health benefit
		I had nothing to lose	Median rank 3[b]	Other
		Doctor advised you	Median rank 3[b]	Physician influence
		Might help others	Median rank 3[b]	Potential benefit to others
		Family advised you	Median rank 5[b]	Other

Continued

Table B.3 Reasons for Participation (*Continued*)

Author	n	Reported reasons for participation	Percent of patients[a]	Reason category assigned by ECRI
Itoh et al.(10)	32	No treatment benefit to myself, but wish to participate anyway	63%	Other
		Trust in doctor	28%	Physician influence[c]
		Advice of doctor	22%	Physician influence[c]
		Some treatment benefit for myself	19%	Potential health benefit[c]
		Better option than no treatment	9%	Potential health benefit[c]
		To help future cancer patients	6%	Potential benefit to others
		Family's advice	0%	Other
Daugherty et al.(11) open-ended	27	Possible therapeutic benefit	85%	Potential health benefit
		Advice or trust in a physician	11%	Physician influence
		Family pressures	4%	Other
		Altruistic reasons	0%	Potential benefit to others
Daugherty et al.(11) closed-ended	27	Possibility of medical benefit	100%	Potential health benefit[c]
		Not having a better option	89%	Potential health benefit[c]
		Trust in institution oncologist	70%	Physician influence[c]
		Trust in institution	67%	Other
		Trust in referring physician	63%	Physician influence[c]
		Trust in institutional oncology nurses	37%	Other
		Wanting to help future cancer patients	33%	Potential benefit to others[c]
		Family wanted it	30%	Other
		To be a part of research	22%	Potential benefit to others[c]

Study	N	Motivation	%	Category
Henzlova et al.(12)	1162	Primary physician recommended	29%	Physician influence
		Contribute to medical science	18%	Potential benefit to others
		Live longer	18%	Potential health benefit
		Help others	10%	Potential benefit to others
		Feel better	12%	Potential health benefit
		Free care and medication	1%	Other
		Other	12%	Other
Wilcox and Schroer(13)	40	Physician influence	47.5%	Physician influence
		Improved health	40%	Potential health benefit
		Coordinator influence	17.5%	Other
		Altruism	15%	Potential benefit to others
		Free care	5%	Other
		Advantage of being closely watched	2.5%	Potential health benefit[c]
		Choice of medication over surgery	2.5%	Potential health benefit[c]
		Friend	2.5%	Other
Mattson et al.(15)	380	Self-directed motivations (medical monitoring, reassurance, physical improvement)	74%	Potential health benefit
		Altruistic motivations (help others, help heart patients, research participation)	65%	Potential benefit to others
		Influence of the medical profession	20%	Physician influence
		Free medical services	16%	Other
		"Harmless"	7%	Other
		Curiosity/"Give it a try"	5%	Other
		Have time available	3%	Other
		Other/Don't know	2%	Other

Continued

Table B.3 Reasons for Participation (*Continued*)

Author	n	Reported reasons for participation	Percent of patients[a]	Reason category assigned by ECRI
Penman et al.(16)	144	Trust in physician	31%	Physician influence
		Physician's information	18%	Physician influence
		It will fight illness	15%	Potential health benefit
		It will cure illness	13%	Potential health benefit
		Will get worse without it	8%	Potential health benefit
		No better treatment	4%	Potential health benefit
		Other physicians agree	3%	Physician influence
		Trust in hospital	1%	Other
		Willing to accept the offer	1%	Other
		Family wanted it	1%	Other
		Consent form information	1%	Other
		Prior treatment same hospital	1%	Other
		Other	1%	Other
		Benefits outweigh risks	0%	Potential health benefit
		To be a part of research	0%	Potential benefit to others
		Prior treatment same physician	0%	Physician influence
		Least expensive	0%	Other
Rodenhuis et al.(17)	10	Hope of improvement of their diseases	50%	Potential health benefit
		Husbands had urged them to go along	30%	Other
		Not able to formulate an explicit motivation	20%	Other

[a]—In some studies, the percentages add to more than 100% because patients were permitted to list more than one reason.

[b]—Henzlova et al.(12) asked patients to rank five reasons in order of importance to the decision. The authors reported only the median rank for each reason.

[c]—Patients in this study were permitted to list more than one reason. Thus, due to the possibility of double-counting patients, we did not add the percentages within any general category. Instead, we used the study's highest relevant percentage as our estimate of the percentage of patients who gave the general reason (see text).

n—Number of patients for whom reasons were reported.

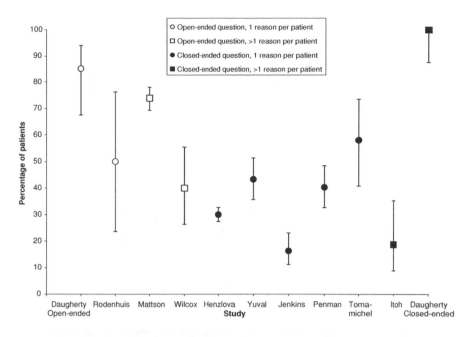

Error bars represent 95% confidence intervals using the Wilson score method. (18)

Figure B.1 Potential Health Benefit as a Reason for Participation.

Some studies permitted each patient to list more than one reason, thus the percentages in the study added to more than 100%. Due to the possibility of counting the results from a given patient more that once (which biases the data towards the reasons given by that patient), we did not add percentages in the aforementioned manner. Instead, for these studies we adopted a conservative approach and used only the highest relevant percentage for the general category. For example, in the study by Itoh et al.(10), 28% of patients cited "trust in doctor" as one of their reasons for participation and 22% cited "advice of doctor" as one of their reasons. Some patients may have cited both of these reasons. To avoid double-counting patients' reasons, we used 28% as the percentage for the general category "physician influence." We used this same process in all other studies that permitted multiple reasons per patient.

Figure B.1 plots the percentages of patients (with 95% confidence intervals) who cited potential health benefit as a reason for participation. The corresponding plots for physician influence and potential benefit to others appear in **Figure B.2** and **Figure B.3**, respectively. These plots demonstrate the wide variability in study results. The range of percentages was 16% to 100% for potential health benefit, 0% to 70% for physician influence, and 0% to 65% for potential benefit to others. We did not include the study by Hutchison(1) in these plots because it employed a ranking method that did not yield

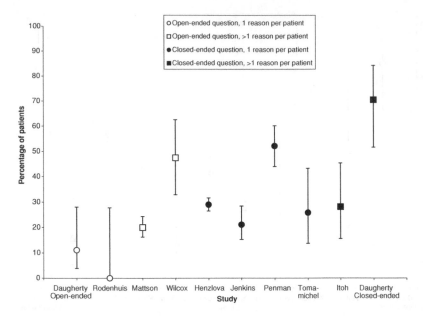

Error bars represent 95% confidence intervals for proportions using the Wilson score method. (18)

Figure B.2 Physician Influence as a Reason for Participation.

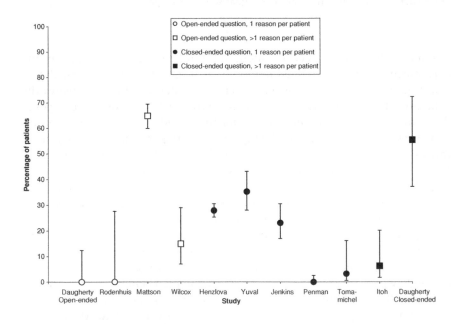

Error bars represent 95% confidence intervals for proportions using the Wilson score method. (18)

Figure B.3 Potential Benefit to Others as a Reason for Participation.

percentages. Daugherty et al.(11) asked both an open-ended question and a closed-ended question, so it appears twice in the figures.

To measure whether the studies reported similar results, we computed a statistic called the Q statistic. This statistic allows one to determine whether the differences among study results ("heterogeneity") are statistically significant. The value of Q increases as the heterogeneity increases. We computed Q separately for each of the three general categories: potential health benefit, physician influence, and potential benefit to others. All three values of Q were statistically significant (388.10 for potential health benefit, 72.48 for physician influence, and 964.25 for potential benefit to others; all p values <0.000001).

These statistically significant values for Q indicate that the percentage of patients who gave these reasons was different in different studies. These differences may have been caused by differences in patient characteristics or study designs. We next investigated seven potential sources of heterogeneity:

- Whether patients had cancer or heart disease
- Average age of patients
- Gender distribution of patients
- Number of patients in the study
- Whether the study used an open-ended format or a closed-ended format
- Whether patients were permitted to cite more than one reason for participation
- Whether patients had been asked about participation in a phase I trial or in a phase II or later trial

To address each of the above potential sources of heterogeneity, we conducted analyses of subgroups. As an example, consider patients' disease as a possible explanation of heterogeneity. We placed the six studies of cancer patients in one subgroup, and the four studies of heart disease patients in another subgroup. Then we computed the Q statistic separately for each subgroup. We performed similar subgroup analyses for each of the other six sources listed above.

In **Table B.4**, the shaded cells indicate subgroups for which there was significant heterogeneity. For example, there was statistically significant heterogeneity among the cancer studies (Q = 93.20, p < 0.000001) as well as among the heart disease studies (Q = 278.40, p < 0.000001) regarding the percentage of patients who cited potential health benefit as a reason for participation. Based on these tests, we conclude that patients' disease was not a sufficient explanation for why the studies' results differed. We drew similar conclusions for the other six sources of heterogeneity because all analyses contained a subgroup of studies with statistically significant heterogeneity. There were some instances in which one of the two subgroups did not have statistically significant heterogeneity. However, in all of these cases, the complementary subgroup did have statistically significant heterogeneity. Therefore, no subgrouping fully eliminated all of the heterogeneity. Based on these results, we conclude that none of the seven potential explanations of heterogeneity are,

Table B.4 Heterogeneity Analyses of Subgroups on Reasons for Participation

Shaded cells indicate subgroups for which there was statistically significant heterogeneity. The p values do *not* refer to significant differences between subgroups. Instead, they refer to heterogeneity of studies *within* a subgroup. See explanation in text.

	Q statistic (p value)[a]		
	Potential health benefit	Physician influence[b]	Potential benefit to others
All studies	388.10 (p < 0.000001)	72.48 (p < 0.000001)	964.25 (p < 0.000001)
Subgroup analyses			
Cancer	93.20 (p < 0.000001)	52.24 (p < 0.000001)	42.71 (p < 0.000001)
Heart disease	278.40 (p < 0.000001)	19.90 (p = 0.000048)	188.50 (p < 0.000001)
Mean age < 58[c]	3.21 (p = 0.73255)	0.41 (p = 0.522061)	150.27 (p < 0.000001)
Mean age ≥58[c]	41.91 (p < 0.000001)	11.65 (p = 0.002951)	4.60 (p = 0.100476)
< 50% female[d]	18.11 (p = 0.000418)	17.95 (p = 0.000451)	4.62 (p = 0.201967)
≥50% female[d]	22.17 (p = 0.000015)	33.18 (p < 0.000001)	42.38 (p < 0.000001)
< 100 patients	42.74 (p < 0.000001)	18.46 (p = 0.001002)	4.85 (p = 0.303012)
≥100 patients	337.75 (p < 0.000001)	52.19 (p < 0.000001)	951.30 (p < 0.000001)
Open-ended	22.27 (p = 0.000057)	17.60 (p = 0.000533)	262.50 (p < 0.000001)
Closed-ended	47.63 (p < 0.000001)	35.27 (p < 0.000001)	428.51 (p < 0.000001)
One reason per patient	99.47 (p < 0.000001)	52.33 (p < 0.000001)	432.82 (p < 0.000001)
More than one reason per patient	65.00 (p < 0.000001)	11.04 (p = 0.004008)	143.57 (p < 0.000001)
Phase I trials	40.60 (p < 0.000001)	6.82 (p = 0.077819)	1.07 (p = 0.784923)
Phase II and later trials	337.76 (p < 0.000001)	57.98 (p < 0.000001)	951.83 (p < 0.000001)

a—For each subgroup, we measured between-study heterogeneity using the Q test. See explanation in text.

b—The percentage of patients who cited physician influence as a reason for participation was reported in all studies except Yuval et al.(9) Thus the overall Q statistic for physician influence was based on 9 studies, whereas the overall Q statistics for potential health benefit and potential benefit to others were each based on 10 studies. The study by Hutchison(1) was not included in any heterogeneity analyses because it reported a unique rank-order methodology.

c—Only five studies of reasons for participation reported the mean or median age of patients. The overall Q statistics for potential health benefit, physician influence, and potential benefit to others were 71.38, 13.71, and 335.39, respectively (all p values < 0.05).

d—Only seven studies of reasons for participation reported the sex distribution of patients. The overall Q statistics for potential health benefit, physician influence, and potential benefit to others were 94.08, 57.30, and 47.94, respectively (all p values < 0.05).

by themselves, sufficient to explain the differences among the results of these studies.

The preceding analyses of subgroups considered only one variable at a time. It would be possible to investigate multiple variables simultaneously in an attempt to explain the large differences between studies' results. For example, patients' disease and patients' age could be used together to account for differences in study results, even though neither variable on its own was sufficient. However, given the relatively small number of studies, we were unable to perform such an analysis.

Despite the heterogeneity between studies, it is informative to estimate the "typical" percentages of patients who gave reasons within the three general categories. These estimates can be reached by combining the results of the studies. A simple average, however, would not be meaningful. As shown by the heterogeneity tests, the studies' outcomes were too different to justify a simple combination of their results. Instead, we performed a more complex computation that was based on a "random effects" statistical model. This calculation allowed us to obtain crude averages in the presence of heterogeneity. We estimated average percentages of 45% for potential health benefit, 27% for physician influence, and 18% for potential benefit to others (see **Figure B.4**).

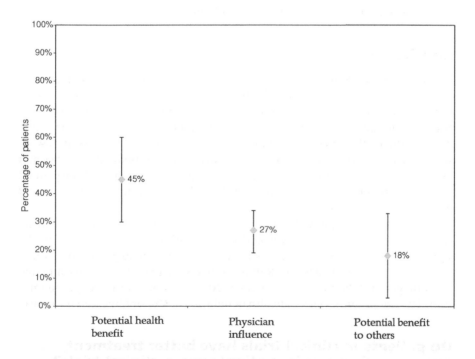

Error bars represent 95% confidence intervals.

Figure B.4 Results of Random-Effects Calculations: Reasons for Participation.

Reasons against participation

Four studies asked patients why they decided not to participate in trials (**Table B.5**). As with the reasons for participation, ECRI assigned a general category to each specific reason in order to permit comparisons between studies. The general categories were: "inconvenience", "concern over experimentation", "potential lack of health benefit", and "physician influence." Another research analyst independently checked the category assignments, and disagreements were resolved through discussion. The category assignments appear in the rightmost column of **Table B.5**. As before, we combined the relevant percentages in studies that permitted only one reason per patient.

The resulting percentages for each of the four categories appear in **Figure B.5**. None of the percentages exceeded 37%, indicating little agreement between patients regarding reasons against participation. As in the section on reasons for participation, we conducted heterogeneity analyses of subgroups in attempting to explain the differences among the results of different studies. However, statistically significant heterogeneity was present in all of the subgroup analyses. To estimate typical percentages of patients citing these reasons against participation, we conducted another set of random-effects calculations (**Figure B.6**). We estimated average percentages of 25% for inconvenience, 20% for concern over experimentation, 19% for potential lack of health benefit, and 14% for physician influence.

Conclusions

Of 14 studies we identified on reasons for participating and not participating in clinical trials, 11 studies cited patients' reasons for participating. These studies reported widely varying results for why patients chose to participate in clinical trials. Although there were differences in patient characteristics and study designs, these differences did not explain why the results of these studies were so different. We used random-effects calculations to combine the studies and estimate the typical percentages of patients who cited reasons in three general categories: potential health benefit (45%), physician influence (27%), and potential benefit to others (18%).

Four studies asked patients why they decided against participation in clinical trials. As with the analyses of reasons for participation, we observed statistically significant heterogeneity in the results that could not be explained by patient characteristics or study designs. Random-effects calculations yielded estimated percentages of 25% for inconvenience, 20% for concern over experimentation, 19% for potential lack of health benefit, and 14% for physician influence.

Do patients in clinical trials have better treatment outcomes than similar patients not in clinical trials?

For patients with a serious or life-threatening illness, a key factor in the decision-making process about trial participation is whether participating will

Table B.5 Reasons Against Participation

Author	n	Reported reasons against participation	Percent of patients[a]	Category assigned by ECRI
Taylor and Leitman(5)	5,972	Belief that they would be better off taking "the standard treatment"	37%	Potential lack of health benefit[b]
		Fear that they might get a placebo rather than actual treatment	31%	Potential lack of health benefit[b]
		Belief that the "standard treatment" would be more effective	30%	Potential lack of health benefit[b]
		Fear of being treated "like a guinea pig"	22%	Concern over experimentation
		Distance they would have to travel to obtain treatment	21%	Inconvenience[b]
		Belief that the cost of treatment would not be covered by insurance	20%	Other
		Amount they would have to pay out-of-pocket	18%	Other
		Fear that their doctor would not be able to choose treatment	18%	Potential lack of health benefit[b]
		The effort involved in the informed consent process	6%	Inconvenience[b]
Jenkins and Fallowfield(6)	51	I trusted the doctor treating me	21.6%	Physician influence
		The idea of randomization worried me	19.6%	Concern over experimentation
		I wanted the doctor to choose my treatment rather than be randomized by a computer	17.6%	Potential lack of health benefit
		Other	41.2%	Other
Ling et al.(7)	196	Patient prefers to wait before entry	17%	Other
		Too unwell/Deterioration in condition	16%	Other
		Lives too far away	11%	Inconvenience
		Patient "didn't want to"/"Not interested"	8%	Other
		Transfer to hospice/hospital/discharge	6%	Inconvenience
		Unable to give informed consent	6%	Other
		Family objection	5%	Other
		Objection to medication	4%	Other
		Not willing/unable to complete forms	3%	Other

Continued

Table B.5 Reasons Against Participation (*Continued*)

Author	n	Reported reasons against participation	Percent of patients[a]	Category assigned by ECRI
		Doctor error/objection	3%	Physician influence
		Too many pills	2%	Other
		Too anxious	2%	Other
		Weekend/evening admission (research nurse unavailable)	1%	Inconvenience
		Placebo fear	1%	Potential lack of health benefit
		Previous participation in trials	1%	Other
		Declined consent reason unknown	17%	Other
Smith and Arnesen(14)	178	Transportation problems	37%	Inconvenience[b]
		Not willing to see other doctors	19%	Physician influence
		Against taking part in experiments	16%	Concern over experimentation
		Insufficient information	11%	Other
		Inconvenient	10%	Inconvenience[b]
		Disliked focusing on disease	8%	Other
		Lack of time	8%	Inconvenience[b]
		Other specified	13%	Other

[a]—In some studies, the percentages add to more than 100% because patients were permitted to list more than one reason.

[b]—Patients in this study were permitted to list more than one reason. Thus, due to the possibility of double-counting patients, we did not add the percentages within any general category. Instead, we used the study's highest relevant percentage as our estimate of the percentage of patients who gave the general reason (see text).

n—Number of patients for whom reasons were reported.

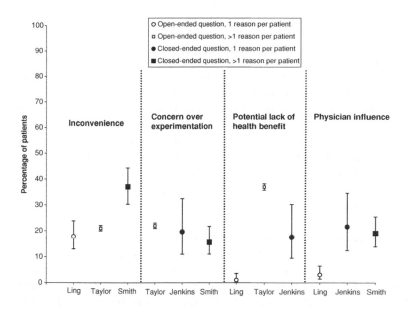

Error bars represent 95% confidence intervals for proportions using the Wilson score method. (18)

Figure B.5 Plot of Reasons Against Participation.

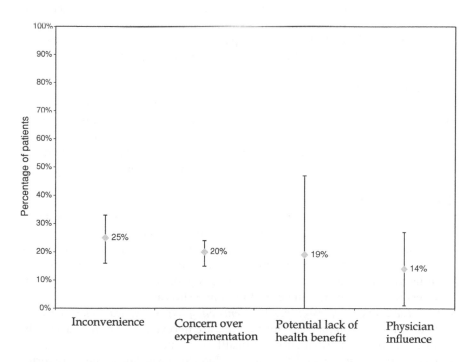

Error bars represent 95% confidence intervals

Figure B.6 Results of Random-Effects Calculations: Reasons Against Participation.

improve the chance of long-term survival and quality of life (QoL). There can be no certain answer to this question, however, because a clinical trial is by definition experimental. Its very existence means that researchers do not know for certain whether the novel treatment has any effect, beneficial or harmful.

Nevertheless, it is possible to examine the health outcomes of the patients who have participated in trials. To place this information in proper context, however, we must also examine the health outcomes of similar patients who were eligible for trials but did not participate in them. It may be informative to compare the health outcomes of patients in these two groups in an attempt to measure the effect of trial participation.

However, there are several potential pitfalls in trying to make this comparison. First, researchers rarely track the progress of patients who did *not* participate in clinical trials. Thus, for most trials, the data are unavailable. Second, clinical trials vary widely in numerous ways (e.g., trial design, patient populations, kinds of treatments), and the effect of participation in past clinical trials may not be generalizable to current or future clinical trials. Third, patients cannot be randomly assigned to either the trial group or the group without trials. Ethically, patients must consent to participate in a clinical trial. Because of the nonrandom assignment, selection biases greatly complicate the comparison of the two groups. For example, if the patients in the trial group were significantly younger than the patients not in trials, then one would expect a priori that the trial group would survive longer. In this situation, it would not be clear whether an observed difference in survival was due to age, trial participation, or both factors.

Despite these pitfalls, we attempted to answer this question by locating trials that compared the health outcomes of patients in each of two groups: patients who participated in a clinical trial, and patients who were eligible for that trial but did not participate. Of particular interest were trials that attempted to control for selection bias when comparing the two groups.

Trial Selection

To be included in analyses of this question, our a priori selection criteria required that a trial meet all of the following inclusion criteria:

- *Include mentally competent patients with an acute or chronic life-threatening illness.* Only trials of life-threatening illnesses were considered because the intended audience for the patient reference guide is patients with a life-threatening illness who are considering enrollment in a clinical trial.
- *Report data for each of two groups of patients: one group in a clinical trial and another group not in any clinical trial.* Both groups are necessary in order to assess the influence of trial participation on health outcomes.
- *Report survival data, quality-of-life data, or both.* Survival data could be reported as survival curves, percentage surviving to a specific time (e.g., three-year survival), and could be reported as either overall survival or disease-free survival. QoL data were considered differently for different diseases.

Table B.6 Excluded Trials

Trial	Reason for exclusion
Cottin et al.(23)	95% of patients in the group not in the trial were not eligible for the trial.
Hjorth et al.(24)	80% of patients in the group not in the trial were not eligible for the trial.
Jha et al.(25)	Authors did not report whether patients in the group not in the trial were eligible for the trial.
Meadows et al.(20)	Nonexperimental research protocols (treatment effectiveness had been established in earlier trials).
Quoix et al.(26)	Some patients in the group not in the trial (unreported percentage) were not eligible for the trial.
Smith and Arnesen(19)	All patients in the trial group had received a placebo, and trial patients who had received the experimental treatment were not reported.
Stiller and Draper(27)	Authors did not report whether patients in the group not in the trial were eligible for the trial.
Stiller and Eatock(28)	Authors did not report whether patients in the group not in the trial were eligible for the trial.

Patient age 18 years or older was not a requirement for this question. The effect of trial participation on children's health outcomes is relevant to an adult's decision about his/her own trial participation because it may reflect widely applicable advantages or disadvantages of being in a trial.

Seventeen trials met the inclusion criteria. Eight of these trials, however, were excluded for reasons listed in **Table B.6**. Six of the excluded trials reported data from a group of nontrial patients in which some patients were not eligible for the trial (or the trial did not report whether patients not in the trial were eligible). Clinical trials often employ stringent inclusion criteria that require a minimum level of health. If patients in the nontrial group were not eligible for the trial, then they might not be comparable to patients in the trial group. Therefore, any differences in posttrial health outcomes between the two groups could be attributed solely to the fact that some patients not in the trial failed the eligibility criteria. The goal of this analysis was to determine the health outcome effects strictly due to trial participation, not to other factors.

Two trials were excluded for other reasons. The trial reported by Smith and Arnesen(19) was excluded because the trial group only included patients who received the placebo arm. As patients decide whether to enter a randomized trial, they do not know which arm of the trial they will be assigned to. Therefore, the overall effect of participating in a trial can only be measured by including data from all arms of that trial, not selected arms. Furthermore, if we examined only the placebo arm, then it would be impossible to measure any effects of the novel treatment, which is the basis for conducting the trial. The trial reported by Meadows et al.(20) was excluded because patients in one group had received research protocols that had already been proven effective. Therefore, these protocols were not experimental, and one would expect a priori that protocol patients would have better health outcomes than other patients who did not receive the protocols due to inadequate access or poor adherence.

Nine trials remained after these exclusions (**Table B.7**). These trials reported on a total of 1,793 patients in trials and 2,654 patients not in trials. The trial by Bertelsen(21) is listed twice in the table because authors reported data separately for each of two trials: one on stage I/II ovarian cancer, and another on stage III/IV ovarian cancer. Therefore, the evidence base consisted of 10 trials. Eight trials investigated cancer patients, and two investigated patients who had heart conditions. Only one trial included children (Lennox et al.(22)). Four trials were conducted in the United States. None of the trials were phase I trials.

Key Study Results

Only survival and QoL were considered for this question. These are the outcomes that are most important to patients. Other outcomes, such as biologic details of cells and cell counts, were not included because they are surrogate outcomes that are only indirectly related to patients' key concerns.

Survival
Reporting of survival included Kaplan-Meier survival curves, and percentage surviving to a specific time point (e.g., three-year survival). Trials were required to report survival for each of the two groups: patients in trials and eligible patients not in trials.

Quality of Life
Because QoL is a subjective concept that was measured differently for different diseases in the trials we examined, we considered each trial separately when assessing QoL. Trials were required to report QoL for each of the two groups.

Results

Survival
As discussed earlier, one problem with comparing the health outcomes of clinical trial patients to those of patients not in trials concerns the potential for selection bias. Because patients cannot be randomly assigned to these groups, there may be important differences in patient characteristics that influence survival. An example in cancer trials is stage of disease: suppose that among

Table B.7 Trial Characteristics

Trial	Disease	Country	Number of trials	Number of patients in trials	Number of patients not in trials	Mean age of trial patients	Mean age of patients not in trials	Percent of females in trials	Percent of females not in trials
Antman et al.(29)	Sarcoma	U.S.	1	42	48	NR	NR	40%	60%
Bertelsen(21)	Ovarian cancer, stage I/II	Denmark	1	72	48	NR	NR	100%	100%
Bertelsen(21)	Ovarian cancer, stage III/IV	Denmark	1	265	96	NR	NR	100%	100%
Boros et al.(30)	Leukemia	U.S.	3	46	46	NR	NR	NR	NR
Brown et al.(31)	Myocardial infarction	U.K.	2	140	329	61.5	64.9	31.4%	33.1%
CASS(32)	Coronary artery disease	U.S.	1	780	1,315	51.2	50.9	9.7%	9.4%
Davis et al.(33)	Nonsmall-cell lung cancer	U.S.	4	78	152	NR	NR	NR	NR
Lennox et al.(22)	Nephro-blastoma	U.K.	1	98	104	NR	NR	NR	NR
Ward et al.(34)	Stomach cancer	U.K.	1	217	493	63[a]	64[a]	30%	31%
Winger et al.(35)	Brain cancer	Canada	1	55	23	52	55	NR	NR
Totals	**Cancer: 8**	**U.S.: 4**	**1: 7**	**1,793**	**2,654**	**56.9**	**58.7**	**52%**	**56%**
	Heart: 2	**U.K.: 3**	**>1: 3**						
		Other: 3							

a—Ward et al.(34) reported median ages

MI—Myocardial infarction; NR—Not reported; U.K.—United Kingdom; U.S.—United States patients in the trial, 30% had advanced metastatic cancer, whereas among eligible patients not in the trial, 60% had advanced metastatic cancer. Obviously, one would expect the average survival of trial patients to be longer than that of patients not in the trial *purely as a result of the different distributions of disease stage*, and not necessarily as a result of trial participation.

To compensate for patient differences, a well-designed trial could use statistical techniques to control for differences in patient characteristics such as disease stage. Ideally, the effect of trial participation on survival would be examined in isolation after factoring out other characteristics that may influence survival. An example of a statistical technique that can achieve this goal is multiple logistic regression. Several predictor variables are used to predict a dichotomous survival outcome (e.g., whether a patient survives for at least four years). Using this technique, it is possible to estimate the *independent* influence of trial participation on survival by simultaneously accounting for other factors.

All 10 trials compared characteristics of patients in trials with patients not in trials (see **Table B.8**). Statistically significant differences were found in 8 of the 10 trials. Of these eight trials, only three used statistical techniques to control for these differences when examining the effect of trial participation on survival. A fourth trial (the Bertelsen(21) trial on stage III/IV ovarian cancer) found that the two groups were not significantly different in any of five patient characteristics. Therefore, in that trial, a comparison of the survival rates of the two groups may be acceptable even without statistically controlling for patient characteristics. A fifth trial (the Davis et al.(33) trial on nonsmall-cell lung cancer) used a "matched control" group in which patients not in the trial were matched to trial patients based on cancer-related prognostic factors.

These five trials are shaded in the table, and they represent the highest-quality trials in our evidence base. We extracted the survival results from these five trials only. Results of other trials were not extracted because it was impossible to determine (based on published reports) whether survival effects were due to trial participation or to significant differences in patient characteristics. In the five extracted trials, survival effects could be attributed solely to trial participation.

The survival results appear in **Table B.9** and **Figure B.7**. Four of the five trials found that patients in trials survived significantly longer than patients not in trials. In another trial, by Brown et al.(31), the difference was in the same direction but was not statistically significant. To provide an appreciation of the size of the survival difference, we estimated three-year overall survival rates for the two groups of patients. This was the only survival outcome reported by one of the trials (Lennox et al.(22)), and we could estimate it from survival curves in three of the other four trials. The range of three-year overall survival was 19% to 80% for patients in trials and 4% to 70% for patients not in trials. We could not conduct heterogeneity analyses of the survival data because authors did not report sufficient data to permit such analyses.

Table B.8 Controls for Differences in Patient Characteristics

Shaded rows indicate trials of highest quality from which we extracted survival data (see explanation in text).

Author	Disease	Which patient characteristics were compared between the groups?	Which showed a significant difference between the groups?	Did the authors control for this characteristic in the survival comparison?	What additional characteristics did the authors control?
Antman et al.(29)	Sarcoma	Age, gender, tumor location & size, stage	Cancer stage	No	None
Bertelsen(21)	Ovarian cancer,I/II	Stage and type of cancer, residual tumor, presence of ascites, tumor cells in ascites	Residual tumor Presence of ascites	No No	None
Bertelsen(21)	Ovarian cancer, III/IV	Stage and type of cancer, residual tumor, presence of ascites, tumor cells in ascites	None	NA	None
Boros et al.(30)	Leukemia	Age, leukocyte count, platelet count, LDH value, uric acid, bilirubin, SGOT findings, performance status, bone marrow cellularity, preleukemic symptoms, fever	Age Leukccyte count	Yes Yes	Platelet count, LDH value, performance status, antibiotics, preleukemic symptoms, fever
Brown et al.(31)	Myocardial infarction	Age, gender, previous MI, previous RV, infarction type, Killip class, management	Age	Yes	Gender, previous MI, type of infarction, Killip class

Continued

Table B.8 Controls for Differences in Patient Characteristics (*Continued*)

Author	Disease	Which patient characteristics were compared between the groups?	Which showed a significant difference between the groups?	Did the authors control for this characteristic in the survival comparison?	What additional characteristics did the authors control?
CASS(32)	Coronary artery disease	Age, gender, race, work status, angina, cigarette use, previous MI, hypertension, congestive failure, diabetes, stroke, peripheral arterial disease, use of nitroglycerin, use of nitrates, use of beta-blockers, use of antiarrhythmic agents, Q-wave MI on ECG, ST depression on ECG, T-wave inversion on ECG, normal ECG, diseased vessels, left-main CA disease, proximal LAD disease, left ventricular score, ejection fraction	Angina Cigarette use Hypertension Diabetes Stroke Use of beta-blockers Q-wave MI on ECG ST depression on ECG Diseased vessels Left-main CA disease Proximal LAD disease	No No No No No No No No No No No	None
Davis et al.(33)	Nonsmall-cell lung cancer	Nodal involvement, tumor size, tumor histology	None	NA	Age, gender, radiation
Lennox et al.(22)	Nephroblastoma	Age, stage of disease	Age	Yes	Stage of disease

Ward et al.(34)	Stomach cancer	Age, gender, symptom duration, disease stage, intent of surgery, residual tumor, metastases, tumor site, number of sites, type of gastrectomy, size of tumor, other pathologic findings	Age	No	None
			Symptom duration	No	
			Tumor site	No	
			Number of sites	No	
			Gastrectomy	No	
			Size of tumor	No	
Winger et al.(35)	Brain cancer	Age, tumor type, performance status	Performance status	No	None

CA—Coronary artery
ECG—Electrocardiogram
LAD—Left anterior descending coronary artery
LDH—Lactic dehydrogenase
MI—Myocardial infarction
NA—Not applicable because the study did not find differences in patient characteristics
RV—Revascularization
SGOT—Serum aspartate aminotransferase

Table B.9 Statistics for Survival Comparison

	Reported survival curves?	Statistical test	Value of test statistic	Confidence interval	Three-year overall survival	
					Percent of patients in trials	Percent of patients not in trials
Bertelsen(21) Stage III/IV	Yes	Mantel-Haenzel test	NR	NR	35%[b]	23%[b]
Boros et al.(30)	Yes	Cox regression slope for trial participation	−0.774[c]	NR	19%[b]	4%[b]
Brown et al.(31)	Yes	Adjusted[a] odds ratio for four-year OS	1.60	0.97–2.63	80%[b]	70%[b]
Davis et al.(33)	No	Relative mortality risk for trial participation	0.39	0.18–0.83	NR	NR
Lennox et al.(22)	No	Adjusted[d] chi square for three-year OS	11.67	NR	77%	58%

[a]—Brown et al.(31) performed a multiple logistic regression in order to adjust for patient characteristics.

[b]—Estimated by ECRI based on published Kaplan-Meier survival curves. One cannot infer the numbers of surviving patients from these percentages due to unreported censoring in the survival data.

[c]—A negative slope in the Cox regression performed by Boros et al.(30) indicated that patients in trials survived longer than patients not in trials.

[d]—Lennox et al.(22) did not report the method of adjustment.

NR—Not reported.

OS—Overall survival.

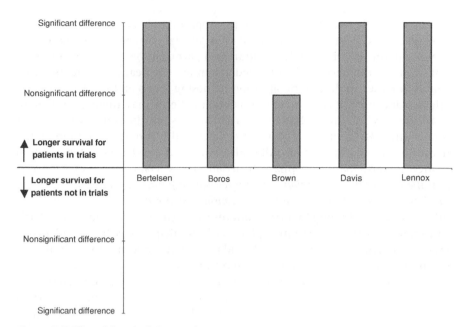

Figure B.7 Plot of Survival Comparison.

Quality of Life

Only 1 of the 10 trials reported QoL outcomes. Brown et al.(31) enrolled patients who had heart attacks, and authors measured the extent of chest pain and breathing difficulty in patients who had participated in clinical trials and patients who had not. However, there were significant differences in pre-study patient characteristics between the groups, and the QoL comparisons did not account for these differences. Thus, one cannot clearly interpret such comparisons within this study.

Conclusions

Based on the available evidence, we conclude that some evidence shows that patients in phase II/III trials survive longer than similar patients who are not in trials. One cannot have great confidence in these results, however, due to the small evidence base.

We identified five trials that controlled for differences in patient characteristics (or found no differences in patient characteristics) when comparing the survival of patients in clinical trials with that of eligible patients not in clinical trials. In four of five trials, patients in trials survived significantly longer than those not in trials.

Only one trial compared the QoL of patients in trials with that of patients not in trials. However, one cannot interpret the results due to differences in patient characteristics between the two groups. Appropriately controlled studies are needed to shed light on the potential effect of trial participation on QoL.

None of the 10 trials analyzed addressed participation in a phase I trial. A phase I trial is not necessarily intended to improve the health of patients in that trial, but rather to determine appropriate dosing levels and measure adverse effects. Of course, it is possible that current patients may themselves benefit from the new treatment, but such an outcome is not the primary intent of a phase I trial. By contrast, a phase II or later trial is intended to improve the health of patients in the trial. All trials in our evidence base for this question related to participation in phase II or later trials. *Consequently, we emphasize that the results for this question are only relevant to patients considering enrollment in phase II or later trials, not to patients considering enrollment in phase I trials.* In other words, the finding that trial patients survived longer in four of five trials cannot be construed by potential phase I trial participants as direct evidence in favor of participation. Instead, we found no evidence relevant to the influence of phase I trial participation on health outcomes.

There are two additional caveats to our results on this subject. Even though some authors controlled for some patient characteristics, one cannot be certain that *all* important characteristics were considered in these trials. There may have been additional characteristics related to survival that were not considered or reported by the authors. Second, statistical significance is an unreliable basis for deciding whether to control for a patient characteristic. Smaller trials are less likely to detect a statistically significant difference between groups. Ideally, a trial would control for patient characteristics *regardless* of whether there were statistically significant differences. However, none of the trials controlled for *all* patient characteristics, and so use of this latter criterion would yield no analyzable trials. Therefore, we extracted data from all trials that attempted to control for observed differences in patient characteristics.

Selected references

1. Hutchison C. Phase I trials in cancer patients: participants' perceptions. Eur J Cancer Care (Engl) 1998 Mar;7(1):15–22.
2. Huizinga GA, Sleijfer DT, van de Wiel HB, van der Graaf WT. Decision-making process in patients before entering phase III cancer clinical trials: a pilot study. Cancer Nurs 1999 Apr;22(2):119–25.
3. Schutta KM, Burnett CB. Factors that influence a patient's decision to participate in a phase I cancer clinical trial. Oncol Nurs Forum 2000 Oct;27(9):1435–8.
4. Searight HR, Miller CK. Remembering and interpreting informed consent: a qualitative study of drug trial participants. J Am Board Fam Pract 1996 Jan-Feb;9(1): 14–22.
5. Taylor H, Leitman R. Misconceptions and lack of awareness greatly reduce recruitment for cancer clinical trials. [article online, Health Care News, Vol. 1, Issue 3]. Rochester (NY): Harris Interactive, Inc.; 2001 Jan 22 [cited 2001 Mar 29]. [3 p]. Available: http://www.harrisinteractive.com.

6. Jenkins V, Fallowfield L. Reasons for accepting or declining to participate in randomized clinical trials for cancer therapy. Br J Cancer 2000 Jun;82(11):1783–8.

7. Ling J, Rees E, Hardy J. What influences participation in clinical trials in palliative care in a cancer centre? Eur J Cancer 2000 Mar;36(5):621–6.

8. Tomamichel M, Jaime H, Degrate A, de Jong J, Pagani O, Cavalli F, Sessa C. Proposing phase I studies: patients', relatives', nurses' and specialists' perceptions. Ann Oncol 2000 Mar;11(3):289–94.

9. Yuval R, Halon DA, Merdler A, Khader N, Karkabi B, Uziel K, Lewis BS. Patient comprehension and reaction to participating in a double-blind randomized clinical trial (ISIS-4) in acute myocardial infarction. Arch Intern Med 2000 Apr 24;160(8): 1142–6.

10. Itoh K, Sasaki Y, Fujii H, Ohtsu T, Wakita H, Igarashi T, Abe K. Patients in phase I trials of anti-cancer agents in Japan: motivation, comprehension and expectations. Br J Cancer 1997;76(1):107–13.

11. Daugherty C, Ratain MJ, Grochowski E, Stocking C, Kodish E, Mick R, Siegler M. Perceptions of cancer patients and their physicians involved in phase I trials. J Clin Oncol 1995 May;13(5):1062–72.

12. Henzlova MJ, Blackburn GH, Bradley EJ, Rogers WJ. Patient perception of a long-term clinical trial: experience using a close-out questionnaire in the Studies of Left Ventricular Dysfunction (SOLVD) Trial. SOLVD Close-out Working Group. Control Clin Trials 1994 Aug;15(4):284–93.

13. Wilcox M, Schroer S. The perspective of patients with vascular disease on participation in clinical trials. J Vasc Nurs 1994 Dec;12(4):112–6.

14. Smith P, Arnesen H. Non-respondents in a post-myocardial infarction trial: characteristics and reasons for refusal. Acta Med Scand 1988;223(6):537–42.

15. Mattson ME, Curb JD, McArdle R. Participation in a clinical trial: the patients' point of view. Control Clin Trials 1985 Jun;6(2):156–67.

16. Penman DT, Holland JC, Bahna GF, Morrow G, Schmale AH, Derogatis LR, Carnrike CL Jr, Cherry R. Informed consent for investigational chemotherapy: patients' and physicians' perceptions. J Clin Oncol 1984 Jul;2(7):849–55.

17. Rodenhuis S, van-den Heuvel WJ, Annyas AA, Koops HS, Sleijfer DT, Mulder NH. Patient motivation and informed consent in a phase I study of an anticancer agent. Eur J Cancer Clin Oncol 1984;20:457–62.

18. Newcombe RG. Two-sided confidence intervals for the single proportion: comparison of seven methods. Stat Med 1998 Apr 30;17(8):857–72.

19. Smith P, Arnesen H. Mortality in non-consenters in a post-myocardial infarction trial. J Intern Med 1990 Sep;228(3):253–6.

20. Meadows AT, Kramer S, Hopson R, Lustbader E, Jarrett P, Evans AE. Survival in childhood acute lymphocytic leukemia: effect of protocol and place of treatment. Cancer Invest 1983;1(1):49–55.

21. Bertelsen K. Protocol allocation and exclusion in two Danish randomised trials in ovarian cancer. Br J Cancer 1991 Dec;64(6):1172–6.

22. Lennox EL, Stiller CA, Jones PH, Wilson LM. Nephroblastoma: treatment during 1970-3 and the effect on survival of inclusion in the first MRC trial. BMJ 1979 Sep 8;2(6190):567–9.

23. Cottin V, Arpin D, Lasset C, Cordier JF, Brune J, Chauvin F, Trillet-Lenoir V. Small-cell lung cancer: patients included in clinical trials are not representative of the patient population as a whole. Ann Oncol 1999 Jul;10(7):809–15.

24. Hjorth M, Holmberg E, Rodjer S, Westin J. Impact of active and passive exclusions on the results of a clinical trial in multiple myeloma. The Myeloma Group of Western Sweden. Br J Haematol 1992 Jan;80(1):55–61.

25. Jha P, Deboer D, Sykora K, Naylor CD. Characteristics and mortality outcomes of thrombolysis trial participants and nonparticipants: a population-based comparison. J Am Coll Cardiol 1996 May;27(6):1335–42.

26. Quoix E, Finkelstein H, Wolkove N, Kreisman H. Treatment of small-cell lung cancer on protocol: potential bias of results. J Clin Oncol 1986 Sep;4(9):1314–20.

27. Stiller CA, Draper GJ. Treatment centre size, entry to trials, and survival in acute lymphoblastic leukaemia. Arch Dis Child 1989 May;64(5):657–61.

28. Stiller CA, Eatock EM. Survival from acute non-lymphocytic leukaemia, 1971-88: a population based study. Arch Dis Child 1994 Mar;70(3):219–23.

29. Antman K, Amato D, Wood W, Carson J, Suit H, Proppe K, Carey R, Greenberger J, Wilson R, Frei E 3d. Selection bias in clinical trials. J Clin Oncol 1985 Aug;3(8):1142–7.

30. Boros L, Chuang C, Butler FO, Bennett JM. Leukemia in Rochester, NY. A 17-year experience with an analysis of the role of cooperative group (ECOG) participation. Cancer 1985 Nov 1;56(9):2161–9.

31. Brown N, Melville M, Gray D, Young T, Skene AM, Wilcox RG, Hampton JR. Relevance of clinical trial results in myocardial infarction to medical practice: comparison of four year outcome in participants of a thrombolytic trial, patients receiving routine thrombolysis, and those deemed ineligible for thrombolysis. Heart 1999 Jun;81(6):598–602.

32. Coronary artery surgery study (CASS): a randomized trial of coronary artery bypass surgery. Comparability of entry characteristics and survival in randomized patients and nonrandomized patients meeting randomization criteria. J Am Coll Cardiol 1984 Jan;3(1):114–28.

33. Davis S, Wright PW, Schulman SF, Hill LD, Pinkham RD, Johnson LP, Jones TW, Kellogg HB Jr, Radke HM, Sikkema WW, Jolly PC, Hammar SP. Participants in prospective, randomized clinical trials for resected non-small cell lung cancer have improved survival compared with nonparticipants in such trials. Cancer 1985 Oct 1;56(7):1710–8.

34. Ward LC, Fielding JW, Dunn JA, Kelly KA. The selection of cases for randomised trials: a registry survey of concurrent trial and non-trial patients. The British Stomach Cancer Group. Br J Cancer 1992 Nov;66(5):943–50.

35. Winger MJ, Macdonald DR, Schold SC, Cairncross JG. Selection bias in clinical trials of anaplastic glioma. Ann Neurol 1989 Oct;26(4):531–4.

Glossary

This glossary covers terms used in this guide and others that are relevant to clinical trials

ABPI (Association of the British Pharmaceutical Industry): The trade association for about a hundred companies in the United Kingdom producing prescription medicines. See http://www.abpi.org.uk.

Adjuvant Therapy is treatment given in addition to the main treatment (for example chemotherapy as well as surgery).

Adverse Drug Reaction (ADR) is an unintended response to a medicinal product, where there is at least a possibility of a causal relationship.

Adverse Event (AE) is an untoward medical occurrence, but there is not necessarily a causal relationship to the treatment or intervention.

Alternative Hypothesis is the hypothesis accepted if the null hypothesis is rejected. It usually states that there is a difference between the interventions.

AMRC (Association of Medical Research Charities) : The AMRC works to advance medical research in the United Kingdom. Its activities focus upon improving the effectiveness of the charitable sector in medical research. See http://www.amrc.org.uk.

Antibodies are blood proteins that are produced by white blood cells when the body recognises that something unfamiliar has got in – for example infecting bacteria. The antibodies attach themselves to the invading bacteria or viruses, which are then destroyed.

Antiemetic is an anti-sickness drug.

Antioxidants are substances that prevent chemical reactions (oxidation) that damage body cells and may lead them to become cancerous.

Baseline Data is information collected on patients at the commencement of a study.

Benign is not cancerous. A benign tumour is a harmless growth that may or may not be operated on.

Best Supportive Care usually refers to the standard (optimal) treatment that a patient may receive.

Bias is a point of view or way of doing things that leads to results that are consistently wrong in one direction or another.

Biopsy is a piece of body tissue taken so that the cells can be examined under a microscope.

Blinding is when one or more parties involved in the trial are kept unaware of the treatment that has been assigned in a trial. Single blinding usually means the participant is unaware, while double blinding means that the participant and research team are all unaware.

Caldicott Guardians are responsible for agreeing and reviewing internal protocols governing the protection and use of patient-identifiable information by staff of their organisations.

Case Control is a type of study that involves identifying patients who have the outcome of interest (cases) and control patients without the same outcome, and looking back to see if they had the exposure of interest.

Case Report Forms (CRFs) are the booklets or folders used to hold the research data.

Case Series is a report on a series of patients with an outcome of interest. No control group is involved.

Causation is when one factor necessarily alters the possibility of a second.

Chromosomes are found in the centre (nucleus) of all human cells. Chromosomes are made of millions of genes (codes that control the cell).

Clinically Relevant Difference is a difference between two interventions that is clinically important.

Clinical Research Associate (CRA) is a representative from either the sponsoring agency or the data collection agency. This individual will 'monitor' the case report forms against the source data and assist in the generation of reports.

Clinical Science is based on observation and treatment of patients (as distinguished from theoretical or basic science).

Clinical Trial is a study in humans intended to discover or verify the effects of a medical intervention (drug, device or procedure), to identify any adverse reactions and to examine its safety and efficacy.

Clinical Trial Units are accredited units that co-ordinate and run large clinical trials.

Cohort Study involves identification of two groups (cohorts) of patients, one that did receive the exposure of interest, and one that did not, and following these cohorts forward for the outcome of interest.

Combination Therapy is the use of two or more types of treatment.

Common Toxicity Criteria (NCI-CTC) are guidelines for grading toxic effects that participants in trials may experience.

Compliance is how closely patients adhere to the treatment or intervention specified in the study protocol.

Confidence Interval is the range of values for a particular variable that indicate that the results are not due to chance.

Confounding Factor is a variable that affects other variables in the study that may result in actual associations being either masked or associations falsely demonstrated.

Continuous Variable is a variable that can be of any possible value along a range.

Control is the term that refers to a participant who does not receive the intervention.

Cost-Benefit Analysis converts effects into the same monetary terms as the costs and compares them.

Cost-Effectiveness Analysis converts effects into health terms and describes the costs for some additional health gain (e.g. cost per additional heart attack prevented).

Cost-Utility Analysis converts effects into personal preferences (or utilities) and describes how much it costs for some additional quality gain.

Crossover Study Design is the administration of two or more experimental therapies one after the other in a specified or random order to the same group of patients.

Cross-Sectional Study is the observation of a defined population at a single point in time or time interval. Exposure and outcome are determined simultaneously.

CT Scan (CAT Scan) is an X-ray scan that creates pictures of the body in cross section

Cyst is a fluid-filled sack or lump.

Cytotoxic treatments are those that are toxic to cells.

Database is a list of information.

Data Fields are spaces in which to record information on records.

Decision Analysis is the application of explicit, quantitative methods to analyse decisions under conditions of uncertainty.

Dependent Variable is a variable whose value depends on one or more other variables – for example blood pressure (dependent variable) can be dependent on obesity (independent variable).

Directorates of Health and Social Care (DHSC): Four Directorates of Health and Social Care (DHSCs) have been established to cover the North, Midlands and

East of England, London and the South of England respectively. The DHSCs support the implementation of government policy by the NHS and Research and Development (R&D), and have a key role to play in underpinning policy development and implementation. See http://www.doh.gov.uk/research/rd3/dhscs.htm.

Distribution is the pattern that values make. Normal distribution is where the pattern of values drawn on a graph is symmetrical.

DNA (Deoxyribonucleic acid). Genes are made of DNA. DNA is the 'genetic code' that controls how cells behave by controlling the type of protein they make.

Dose Response is the amount of the investigated treatment needed to engender the desired response in the participant.

Early Stopping is when a trial is halted before its planned completion because of identified adverse or beneficial effects.

Effectiveness refers to how well the intervention has worked in patients that were offered it.

Efficacy refers to whether the intervention worked or not in those patients who received it.

Endpoint is a study outcome measure.

Enzymes are proteins that control chemical reactions in the body.

Epithelial Tissue is skin tissue that covers the outside and inside of the body. It covers all the body organs, and lines all the tubes and cavities of the body. Cancers of epithelial tissue are called carcinomas.

Equipoise is a state of true uncertainty on the part of a researcher about which intervention will achieve a better outcome.

Ethics Committee is a group of professional and consumer experts that review the ethical considerations of research involving human participants. All clinical research must be submitted to this committee and approval sought before the research can begin.

Evidence-Based Healthcare extends the application of the principles of *Evidence-Based Medicine* (see below) to all professions associated with healthcare, including purchasing and management.

Evidence-Based Medicine is the conscientious, explicit and judicious use of current best evidence in making decisions about the care of individual patients. The practice of evidence-based medicine means integrating individual clinical expertise with the best available external clinical evidence from systematic research.

Excess Treatment Cost is the difference between the treatment costs incurred as a result of a particular piece of R&D and those that would have been incurred had the patients concerned been receiving the standard alternative service. Excess treatment costs only arise where experimental services are being provided, or where standard care is being provided in a different way or location compared to routine practice.

Exclusion refers to the situation where disproportionate numbers of discrete groups of patients are not included in the study population.

Exclusion Criteria are specified restrictive controls on the recruitment of particular patient sub-groups that are not eligible to participate in the study.

Factorial Design is a type of study that can show the effect of two (or more) interventions independently and their interaction. If two drugs were being compared, the four arms of the study would be Placebo A + Placebo B; Drug A + Placebo B; Drug B + Placebo A; Drug A + Drug B.

Feasibility Study is a small preliminary study to assess the practicalities of doing a larger study. It is also called a *Pilot Study*.

First-Line Treatment is the preferred therapy for a given condition.

Follow-Up Data is information collected after patients have been entered into a trial.

GAfREC (Governance Arrangements for Research Ethics Committees) : A standard framework for the process of review of the ethics of all proposals for research in the NHS and Social Care. It sets out general standards and principles for an accountable system of research ethics committees, working collaboratively to common high standards of review and operating process throughout the NHS. See http://www.doh.gov.uk/research/documents/gafrec.doc.

Genes are coded messages that tell cells how to behave and so control the body's growth and development. Genes are made of DNA and are grouped to make chromosomes.

Good Clinical Practice (GCP) is a systematically developed statement designed to assist practitioners and patients make decisions about appropriate healthcare in specific clinical circumstances. The development of these guidelines is based on the World Medical Association Declaration of Helsinki.

Good Manufacturing Practice (GMP) is a set of guidelines to ensure medicinal products are manufactured, packaged and labelled to agreed standards.

Historical Controls are groups of patients treated in the past that are used as comparisons in the present.

Hormone Therapy is treatment for a disease with hormones or blocking the action of hormones.

HTA (Health Technology Assessment): HTA is one of the three main national programmes funded from the NHS R&D levy, the others being New and Emerging Applications of Technology (NEAT) and Service Delivery and Organisation (SDO). The purpose of the HTA programme is to ensure that high-quality research information on the cost, effectiveness and broader impact of health technologies is produced in the most efficient way for those who use, manage and provide care in the NHS. 'Health technologies' include all devices, equipment, drugs and procedures across all sectors of healthcare and is not confined to new drugs or pieces of sophisticated equipment. See http://www.hta.nhsweb.nhs.uk/.

Human Tissue Authority (HTA): The Human Tissue Authority will replace the Retained Organs Commission, due to close on 31 March 2004. The authority will oversee the use of human tissue for anatomical examination, education and training related to human health and research, research and transplantation. Any person carrying out these activities must be licensed and there are strict guidelines and procedures governing the use of tissue to be used for donation or research purposes. See http://www.wellcome.ac.uk/en/genome/geneticsandsociety/hg15n020html.

Hyperplasia is increased cell growth, but the cells are normal.

Inclusion Criteria define the particular patient sub-groups that are eligible to take part in the study.

Independent Data Monitoring Committee (IDMC) is a committee that at intervals looks at the progress of a trial, the safety data and endpoints. It can recommend whether the trial should be continued, modified or stopped.

Independent Variable is a variable whose value influences one or more other variables – for example obesity (independent variable) can influence blood pressure (dependent variable) on.

Informed Consent is the process that provides information to a patient so the patient can make a choice or state a preference about the treatment offered.

Interaction is when one variable affects other variables differently (for example the effects of a drug may be different in males and females).

Interval Data are data classified into equal intervals – for example temperature. It does not mean that 20° is twice as hot as 10°.

Intervention is the diagnostic, treatment or device under investigation.

Investigational Product is the product being tested or used as a reference in a clinical trial.

Investigator is the person who has overall responsibility for the recruitment and data handling within a centre. This person may be called the principal investigator, chief investigator, lead investigator or local investigator. This may depend on the overall role of the investigator within the trial. The investigator is usually a qualified medical practitioner and has a role that includes a clinical obligation as well as a scientific commitment.

Involve (formerly Consumers in NHS Research) aims to ensure that consumer involvement in R&D in the NHS, Public Health and Social Care improves the way that research is prioritised, commissioned, undertaken and disseminated. See http://www.invo.org.uk/.

Legally Acceptable Representative is an individual, or other body.

Life-Table Analysis is a graph where the progress of a patient is plotted against time.

Lost to Follow-Up is when patients can no longer be followed up for the planned period of time.

Lymphatic System is a system of tubes and glands in the body that filters body fluid and fights infection.

Malignant is cancerous. The opposite of benign.

Marker is a chemical substance produced by a cancer and used to monitor the progress of the disease. It is usually measured by a blood test.

Maximum Tolerated Dose (MTD) is the largest dose of a medicinal product that has been found, usually from phase I and II trials, to be safe in humans.

Mean is another term for the average.

Median (or middle value) is when for a group of values, one half of the values is higher than the median, and one half is lower.

Meta-Analysis is a quantitative method of pooling data from many studies to reach a summary estimate of effect for a body of literature.

Meta Register: The *meta* Register of Controlled Trials is a free, searchable, international database of more than 14 000 ongoing randomised controlled trials in all areas of healthcare. At present, the *m*RCT also contains some completed trials. See http://www.controlled-trials.com/.

MRC (Medical Research Council) : The UK MRC is a national organisation funded by the UK Government. It promotes research into all areas of medical and related science and is independent in its choice of which research to support, though it does work in close partnership with Health Departments, other Research Councils, industry and others to identify and respond to current and future health needs. See http://www.mrc.ac.uk/.

MRI (Magnetic Resonance Imaging) is a scan that uses magnetism to build up a picture of the organs inside your body.

Mode is the most common value in a group.

Monitoring is the process of overseeing the conduct of a trial, ensuring it complies with Good Clinical Practice (GCP).

Multi-centre is when things are done in more than one centre or place.

Multi-Disciplinary Team (MDT): The MDT is a group of healthcare professionals from a variety of backgrounds who meet in the hospital to discuss patients' treatment and care before they see those patients in the clinics. It is often at the MDT meeting that patients who may be eligible to take part in clinical research are identified.

Multiple Comparisons are when two or more treatment comparisons involving the same outcome measure are made at the same time point.

Mutation is a change in a gene. If a gene is mutated, the protein it makes will be abnormal. It can also alter how a gene works.

Myeloma is a cancer that develops from the plasma cells of bone marrow.

Negative Control is when patients in a trial receive inactive control treatment.

NELH (National Electronic Library for Health): This website is a digital library designed for NHS staff, patients and the public. See http://www.nelh.nhs.uk. The website has a section about how clinical trials work and what people may expect if they are asked to take part in a trial. The section was developed with patients and members of the public, and is designed for people in the United Kingdom who might be asked to take part in a clinical trial during the course of their healthcare. This section does not provide information about specific trials. See http://www.nelh.nhs.uk/clinicaltrials/.

NHS R&D Forum: The NHS Research and Development Forum is an organisation for individuals and departments involved in the management and planning of R&D activities and in conducting R&D in health and social care. The purpose of the forum is to improve the environment for research within organisations delivering health and social care by encouraging high standards and providing support and communication networks. The forum is an inclusive organisation open to all involved in R&D, including directors, managers, administrators, consumers and researchers themselves. The activities of the forum encompass research across the full range of health and social care including community and primary care, secondary and tertiary care, public health and social services. See http://www.rdforum.nhs.uk/.

NICE (National Institute for Clinical Excellence): NICE was set up as a Special Health Authority for England and Wales on 1 April 1999. It is part of the National Health Service (NHS), and its role is to provide patients, health professionals and the public with authoritative, robust and reliable guidance on current 'best practice'. The guidance will cover both individual health technologies (including medicines, medical devices, diagnostic techniques and procedures) and the clinical management of specific conditions. It is based in London. See http://www.nice.org.uk.

Nominal Data are data in unordered categories – for example male and female.

Null Hypothesis is the hypothesis accepted if the alternative hypothesis is rejected. It usually states that there is no difference between the interventions.

Number Needed to Treat is the number of patients who need to be treated to prevent one bad outcome.

Oncologist is a doctor whose specialty is the treatment of cancer.

Ordinal Data are data in ordered categories – for example mild, moderate, severe.

Outcomes are measurements of change occurring as a result of an intervention. An example of an outcome is the time of disease-free survival after receiving an investigational compound.

Parallel Group Design is the most common trial design where participants are allocated, usually randomly, to receive a particular intervention, and the results of the interventions compared.

PCTs (Primary Care Trusts): PCTs are free-standing, legally established, statutory NHS bodies that are accountable to their health authority. PCTs have responsibility for securing the provision of the fuller range of services for the local populations. They have responsibility for all family health services practitioners allowing a coherent view of the development of all NHS services in the area. PCTs have responsibility for the management, development and integration of all primary care services including medical, dental, pharmaceutical and optical services. See http://www.doh.gov.uk/pricare/pcts.htm.

Pharmacodynamic is the action of a drug in the body over a period of time.

Pharmacokinetic is the way a drug is processed in the body over a period of time.

Phase I, II and III Trials are terms to describe the different types of trials used during the evaluation of a new drug or treatment. Phase I and II trials are not usually randomised and are often concerned with assessing toxicity and dose response. If the effects of the new drug or therapy appear to be positive, phase III trials are conducted. These trials are usually RCTs with the new treatment compared against the existing treatment. If there is no standard treatment it may be compared with a placebo, or 'best supportive care'.

Phase IV is a type of study usually conducted after the new therapy has been approved for marketing. This type of study often focuses on adverse events in the clinical setting and is not normally a controlled trial.

Pilot Study is a small preliminary study to assess the practicalities of doing a larger study. It is also called a *Feasibility* study.

Placebo is a treatment with no pharmacological or physiological effect. There may be a psychological effect.

Population is the group of people being studied.

Power is the probability that the differences in effects found in a research study are not due to chance.

Pre-clinical usually refers to stages of research done before testing on humans.

Pre-randomisation is the process of seeking consent for the particular therapy offered and not discussing the underlying random allocation of treatment.

Primary Cancer/Tumour is where the cancer started. The type of cell that has become cancerous will be the primary cancer – for example if a biopsy from the liver or lung contains cancerous breast cells, then the primary cancer is breast cancer.

Primary Endpoint is the most important outcome measure in a study.

Prognosis is the likely outlook (in terms of cure or control) for someone with a disease.

Prospective Follow-Up Study is a study where patients with specific characteristics are identified and followed up.

Protocol: A protocol is a formally written, step-by-step guide to the study. It should include all of the appropriate information for the study. A well-designed and well-written protocol should provide anyone new reading it with all the operational information to run the study.

Qualitative is a way of expressing something without numbers.

Quantitative is a way of expressing something with numbers.

Randomisation is the process of assigning trial participants to treatment or control groups using an element of chance to reduce bias.

Randomised Controlled Trials (RCTs): There are many different types of RCTs. The most common types used in clinical trials are designed around whether or not the investigators and participants know which intervention is being assessed.

Random Permuted Blocks is when a number of treatments are randomly sequenced – for example three treatments could be given in the order ABC, ACB, BAC, CAB, CBA.

Range is the difference between the smallest and the biggest value.

Raw Data are the measurements and observations before they have been processed or analysed.

Recurrence is cancer that has returned after treatment.

Reliability is the consistency of measures over time.

Research and Development (R&D) Costs are one of three categories into which the costs of externally funded non-commercial R&D can be divided (the other two are Service Support Costs and Treatment Costs). R&D costs are the costs of the R&D itself and are met by the research funder. They include the costs of data collection and analysis and other activities needed to answer the question being addressed. They can include pay and indirect costs of staff employed to carry out the R&D.

Sample Size is the number of patients needed in a study to make a statistically significant result likely in a given period.

Sarcoma is cancer that has arisen in connective tissue (for example muscle, bone or nerves).

Screening is the process of determining if individuals meet certain criteria. This may be done to see if patients are eligible to take part in a study.

Secondary Cancer (Metastasis) is cancer that has spread. Cancer cells have broken away from the primary cancer (where the cancer began) and spread to another part of the body where they have begun to grow. Secondary cancer is treated according to the type of cells it is made up of. For example, breast cancer cells that spread to the lung will respond to breast cancer treatments, not lung cancer treatments, because they are breast cancer cells no matter where they are growing.

Secondary Endpoint(s) are less important outcome measures in a study other than the primary endpoint.

Selection Bias is an error that occurs if the characteristics of participants taking part in a study are different from those not taking part.

Serious Adverse Event (SAE) or Serious Adverse Drug Reaction (Serious ADR) is any medical occurrence that requires hospitalisation, is life-threatening, or results in significant disability/incapacity or death.

Service Support Costs are one of three categories into which the costs of externally funded non-commercial R&D can be divided (the other two are R&D Costs and Treatment Costs). These costs are the *additional* patient care costs associated with the research, which would end once the R&D activity in question had stopped, even if the same patient care service continued to be provided.

Significance Level (P Value) is a pre-set probability level at which it is agreed that the null hypothesis will be rejected. It is typically set at 5%. This means there is a 19 in 20 probability that the results are significant.

Site File is the document used to store all of the material that is not patient data which is relevant to the study. This will include all study correspondence together with copies of CVs of the research team. It is important that all correspondence is kept and filed in a logical order usually chronological.

Source Data refers to the original recording of data of a patient. This may be part of the patient case records or notes.

Sponsor is an individual, company, institution or organisation that takes responsibility for the initiation, management and/or financing of a clinical trial.

Standard Treatment is the accepted, routine treatment for a given disease or condition.

Stratification is a way of randomising participants while at the same time keeping particular groups together – for example there may be separately randomised groups of males and females to ensure there is a balance of sexes in the study.

Study Arm is one part of a study. Patients in different arms are randomised to receive different treatments.

Sub-Group is a separate part of the study population – for example all females over 60 years of age.

Suspected Unexpected Serious Adverse Reactions (SUSAR) are all suspected adverse reactions related to an investigational medicinal product (IMP) that are unexpected and serious.

Therapeutic Study is a trial of an intervention that may have clinical benefit.

Toxicity refers to the undesired effects of the treatment under investigation.

Treatment Costs are one of three categories into which the costs of externally funded non-commercial R&D can be divided (the other two are Service Support Costs and R&D Costs). Treatment costs are the patient care costs that would continue to be incurred if the patient care service in question continued to be provided after the R&D activity had stopped. Where patient care is being provided which differs from the normal, standard treatment for that condition (either an experimental treatment or a service in a different location from where it would normally be given), the difference between the total treatment costs and the costs of the 'standard alternative' (if any) can be termed the *Excess Element of Treatment Costs* (or just *Excess Treatment Costs*), but is nonetheless part of the Treatment Cost, not a Service Support or R&D Cost.

Treatment Difference/Treatment Effect is the difference measured by one of the study endpoints between the groups in the study.

Tumour is a cancerous lump.

Ultrasound is a scan using sound waves to build up a picture of the inside of the body.

Unblinding is when the treatment assignments of trial participants is revealed to those groups who until that point had been denied this information.

Unexpected Adverse Drug Reaction is an adverse reaction not consistent with the product information.

Validity is the extent to which a measure really measures the concept that it purports.

Variable is any measurement or characteristic recorded in a trial.

Variance is the degree to which a set of quantities varies.

Washout is a period of time in a trial when a participant receives no study medication.

White Blood Cells are cells in the blood that fight infection and produce antibodies.

Index

Printed and bound by CPI Group (UK) Ltd, Croydon, CR0 4YY

27/10/2024

14580383-0004